Overcoming Common Problems Series

D0994016

Overcoming Common Problems Series

Overcoming Common Problems

Epilepsy
Complementary and alternative treatments

DR SALLIE BAXENDALE

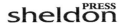

First published in Great Britain in 2012

Sheldon Press
36 Causton Street
London SW1P 4ST
www.sheldonpress.co.uk

The author and publisher have made every effort to ensure that the external website
and email addresses included in this book are correct and up to date at the time of
going to press. The author and publisher are not responsible for the content, quality or
continuing accessibility of the sites.

British Library Cataloguing-in-Publication Data
A catalogue record for this book is available from the British Library

ISBN 978–1–84709–154–3
eBook ISBN 978–1–84709–230–4

Typeset by Caroline Waldron, Wirral, Cheshire
First printed in Great Britain by Ashford Colour Press
Subsequently digitally printed in Great Britain

Produced on paper from sustainable forests

'There is scarcely a substance in the world capable of passing through the gullet of a man that has not, at one time or another, enjoyed the reputation of being anti epileptic.'

Sir Edward Henry Sieveking (1850)

Contents

Foreword

All over the world, complementary and alternative approaches to epilepsy therapy are widely used. In a survey from the USA in 2003, for instance, 44 per cent of patients with epilepsy had used some form of alternative treatment, and similar numbers are found in studies from other countries. However, many doctors practising orthodox medicine take the view that it is unclear how useful such therapies are likely to be, because the standard of evaluation is poor. The situation is complicated by the large and diverse range of potential treatments, and the sometimes excessive claims made for them by unscrupulous practitioners, some of whom have a financial stake in their treatments. Some of the therapies have a theoretical basis to explain their use, but in others there is no such underpinning. In spite of all this, the therapies remain popular and sometimes effective. I recall many of my own patients opting for treatments which, superficially, seemed futile and pointless, and yet were for some highly successful. For others, though, the treatments were ineffective and their use demoralizing and expensive. The popularity of alternative treatments is perhaps not surprising when one considers that conventional medical therapy is also sometimes ineffective and cannot 'cure' epilepsy. In any chronic medical condition, the search for effective remedies will not, and should not, be confined to orthodox medicines.

The assessment of the role of these treatments is complicated by the fact that many practitioners of alternative medicine renounce a scientific approach to evaluation as meaningless. Of course, there is some truth in the view that inflexible scientific assessment will often overlook the more complex or subtle aspects of therapy, and that scientific rigour has a tendency to dehumanize individual experience. Nevertheless, unless a punctilious and thorough approach is taken, the evaluation of therapy can be distorted and biased. On the other hand, many conventional doctors, when asked by patients if this or that alternative therapy might be helpful, will be dismissive – and sometimes patronizing – an attitude born largely of ignorance.

Where can any person – patient or doctor – turn to for information in this area which has proved such a minefield? Although much is written on the internet, it is frequently biased and at times frankly misleading, and it is difficult to know what to trust and what to believe. This is where this book comes in. It aims to provide, as no other has, a balanced evaluation of a range of alternative and complementary therapies, in a scientific manner yet keeping the scientific approach in perspective, and with a strong emphasis on the actual objective experiences of patients. This is a difficult balancing act, and yet Dr Baxendale has achieved this in an outstandingly successful manner. Many therapies are considered, including stress reduction, diet, physical, psychological, herbal, traditional and modern treatments. The format of the book is interesting. For each therapy, the objective evidence and theoretical basis is considered in turn, and then useful practical information given. Each is summarized and advice given on the question, 'Will this work for you?' The book gives an account which is full of wisdom and, unlike many writings in this area and in medicine generally, it is mercifully free of jargon. The text is lucid and wonderfully precise and can be easily understood.

Sallie Baxendale is a psychologist with a highly rated international reputation for her work in epilepsy. She has made many original and innovative contributions, and has also had a long-standing interest in alternative and innovative ways to tackle the condition. Indeed, she is one of the few authorities in the world who can write usefully on this topic, and she is to be congratulated on producing a unique and valuable book, which should be read by all patients who wish to explore these therapeutic avenues, and indeed all doctors who are asked to advise on these treatments. I know of no better, clearer or more authoritative text in this complex and important area.

Professor Simon Shorvon
Professor of Neurology, Institute of Neurology
University College London

Acknowledgements

Without the time and very practical support of John Kirby and Wendy Baxendale I could not have completed this book. Thanks are also due to Matilda and Georgia Kirby who, in a variety of ways, gave up their time as well. I am also grateful to Mr Julian Rowe-Jones, who cleared the way along the course of this project.

I am indebted to Profs Schachter, Pacia and Devinsky, whose previous work in this area proved a valuable resource in my research for this book. I had help, too, from my friends and colleagues at the National Hospital for Neurology, London. In particular, I would like to thank Dr Pamela Thompson whose quiet patience and support have been invaluable, not just during the writing of this book, but throughout my career. Finally, I would like to thank my editor, Fiona Marshall, whose enthusiasm for epilepsy and belief in this book enabled me to write it.

Note to the reader

This book is not intended to replace advice from your doctor. Consult your pharmacist or doctor if you believe you have any of the symptoms described, and if you think you might need medical help.

1

Introduction

What is epilepsy?

Everything we do, from walking down the road to completing the most complex puzzle, requires our brain cells to communicate effectively with each other. When we are born, many of the connections between these cells have yet to be made. As babies learn to coordinate their bodies, they gain control over their actions. The changes in the brain that happen to allow this control are immense, with billions of brain cells establishing rapid connections with each other. These connections do not just enable us to physically control our bodies, they are essential for learning and remembering things too. Our brain cells need to communicate with each other in a rapid, effective and ordered way, to enable us to carry out even the simplest task. With over 100 billion brain cells involved, the human brain is one of the most complex systems on the planet.

Given this complexity, it is not surprising that sometimes the system breaks down. When the cells in parts of the brain begin to communicate with each other in a disordered way, a seizure can occur. The nature of the seizure will depend on which parts and how much of the brain is involved. This is why seizures can look and feel so dissimilar for different people. If only small parts of the brain begin to communicate with each other in a disordered way, the person may simply experience an odd smell or a sensation of tummy butterflies. What you feel depends entirely on which part of the brain is not working correctly. A feeling of déjà vu (intense familiarity, like it has all happened before) is common for people if parts of the memory system within the brain are involved in the disturbance. Others may experience intense feelings of anxiety or even terror that appear out of the blue, if the 'fear' centres within the brain are affected. Disordered communications between brain cells can also cause physical effects, ranging from an uncontrollable urge to giggle, to nausea, sometimes even vomiting. These small seizures have been given various labels over the years, including auras and simple partial seizures. The current terminology recommended by the International League Against Epilepsy (ILAE) for these attacks is 'focal seizures without impairment of consciousness or awareness'.

If larger areas of the brain are involved in a seizure, a person may lose awareness. Losing awareness is different to losing consciousness. A person who is unconscious is inert and immobile. People who lose awareness during a seizure may still walk around, gesture and even talk; nevertheless, they are not completely aware of their surroundings. They may respond automatically to some of the things or people they encounter during the seizure. These behaviours might include pouring water from a jug (with no cup present) or picking up a telephone when it has not rung. Fiddling with clothes and even completely undressing can occur during these kinds of seizures. These types of seizures can be some of the most dangerous as some people cannot perceive danger or respond to pain while the brain is behaving in this way.

All epilepsy doctors have encountered people who have sustained very severe, often life-threatening injuries during these seizures.

Karen
Karen, a young mother, was cooking chips at teatime for her young children when she experienced a focal seizure. She placed her right hand into the chip pan full of boiling oil during the seizure and left it there for over a minute. Most of the flesh had burnt off by the time the seizure ended.

John
John, who has had poorly controlled epilepsy since childhood, has been hit by a bus, not once – but twice! On both occasions, on his way to hospital appointments, he walked out into traffic, oblivious to the oncoming vehicles.

These injuries serve as sobering reminders of the dangers associated with epilepsy. Even something as simple as making a cup of tea can result in severe injuries, if an individual experiences one of these seizures during the task. As with simple partial seizures and auras these seizures have been classified under different names in the past including 'petit mal' or 'complex partial seizures'. In this book we will call these seizures 'focal seizures with impaired awareness', following the most recent recommendations of the ILAE.

If very large areas of the brain are involved in a seizure it is classified as a 'generalized seizure'. In these attacks, the person experiencing the seizure will drop to the floor. In a 'drop attack', recovery is almost immediate. In a generalized 'tonic-clonic seizure', the muscles of the body contract rhythmically, leading to a shaking appearance. This is not just evident in the arms and legs, but in the facial muscles too. People can often be incontinent during these seizures. Although 'foaming at the mouth' is frequently associated with these types of attack in the public imagination, this is in fact incorrect. People may produce excessive saliva during the attack, but the 'foaming' seen in artistic representations of seizures firmly belongs in the realm of the supernatural.

Fortunately, in the vast majority of seizures, the brain recognizes that regular communications have been disrupted and it strives to re-establish normality. As a result most seizures are self-limiting, that is they run their own course without any outside intervention. It is very rare that seizures of any kind last more than five minutes. Sometimes, people can experience a run of seizures, one after another with very little recovery time in between, and these can look to the observer like one very long seizure. More rarely, the brain's own seizure shut-down mechanism can malfunction and a seizure can continue without stopping. This is called 'status epilepticus' and is the most serious kind of seizure. Someone in status epilepticus requires prompt medical attention and if left untreated it can result in brain damage or even death.

Many different reasons

There are many different reasons why people have seizures. For some, seizures are the result of brain damage that occurs following an accidental head injury. Brain infections such as meningitis and encephalitis can also lead to seizures. Tumours which grow in the brain can also disrupt the communication pathways within the brain and result in epilepsy. For others, something may have happened very early on when they were developing in the womb to cause their brains to develop in an abnormal way. For most of these people, magnetic resonance imaging (MRI) scans can reveal the areas of damage or abnormal development that may be responsible for setting off seizure activity within the brain. Metabolic disorders and some genetic conditions can also be associated with epilepsy. However, for a dwindling percentage of people, the doctors can find no obvious reason why the brain malfunctions in this way. Since 2010, these people are classified by the ILAE as having 'epilepsy of unknown cause'. These conditions used to be called 'idiopathic' or 'cryptogenic' epilepsies (cryptogenic means hidden). All that these terms really mean is that medical science cannot yet explain why these people have seizures. People who would have been given a diagnosis of cryptogenic epilepsy ten years ago may have areas of damage or abnormality within their brains that can now be seen clearly on the latest scans. New genetic conditions associated with epilepsy are also being discovered every year. Hidden brain abnormalities in people who are given a diagnosis of epilepsy of unknown cause today may become apparent in the near future as medical scans and technologies advance.

Seizure thresholds are based on the idea of a dam with water building up behind it. When the water gets too high behind the dam, it is breeched and the water flows over the top. This breech represents a seizure. Just as there are many factors that can contribute to the high water levels behind a dam, there are also many factors that can lead to a theoretical 'breech' in brain function leading to a seizure. Everyone has a seizure threshold. However, most people are never in the situation where their threshold is exceeded and so they never have a seizure. But for people with recurrent seizures, their natural threshold seems to be set at a lower level than other people. A combination of factors appears to lead to regular breechings of this threshold, resulting in seizures.

Because there are many different reasons why people have seizures, epilepsy can affect people of all ages. As a general rule of thumb, epilepsy is more common in children than in adults. The prevalence of the condition rises again in the elderly population, where seizures may be the result of other illnesses that affect brain function, including strokes and cerebral vascular disease.

Conventional medical treatments

Anti-epileptic drugs are an effective way of controlling seizures for the majority of people with epilepsy. Some people find that a low dose of a single drug works well for them. Their seizures stop and they are able to return to a full life. For instance, this recovery may include a return to car driving a year after their last seizure. For others, it may take a combination of drugs and they may need to take four or five different medications in the morning and again in the evening to completely control their seizures. Unfortunately, the right combination of drugs can have side effects. These can include rashes, weight gain, unwanted facial hair, drowsiness and difficulties in concentration. Living with these side effects can, occasionally, be more problematic than the actual seizures for some people. Getting the balance right between good seizure control and minimal side effects can sometimes take the doctor and person with epilepsy many years of trial and error to achieve. Unfortunately, for approximately 30 per cent of people with epilepsy, no combination of drugs is completely effective and they continue to experience seizures despite taking the maximum dose of many anti-epileptic drugs, morning, noon and night.

Why consider complementary treatments?

People may consider complementary and alternative treatments for epilepsy for many reasons. Some may have reached the end of the road in the medical options available to them. If the drugs do not work, surgery may be possible for a small minority of people, but surgery is not an option for most people with epilepsy. Other people may have a sensitivity to the drugs offered, meaning they cannot tolerate the doses needed to get the best seizure control. Others may instinctively dislike the idea of a lifelong dependence on medication and may wish to get the maximum possible benefit from treatments they perceive to be more gentle, working with natural rhythms of their body. Whatever the motivation, it is clear that increasing numbers of people with epilepsy are now looking beyond just taking pills to help them live with their condition.

The aim of this book

For anyone looking for information on complementary treatments for epilepsy, nowadays the internet is often the first point of call. Unfortunately, much of the information on the web is written by people who have a vested interest in selling their product or approach to you. The glowing testimonials of 'miracle cures' on many websites are, at best, anecdotal and, at worst, simply fictitious. It is difficult to know who to trust on the internet. The purpose of this book is to present the objective scientific evidence for and against some of the most popular complementary treatments for epilepsy available today. Hopefully, it will give you some ideas as to what might work for you, and will save you time and money in ruling out the approaches that are unlikely to help.

How to use this book

Chapter 2 presents the criteria against which the complementary treatments presented in this book have been judged and gives some guidance as to how you can evaluate whether a new treatment is really working for you. Some treatments may be effective for some kinds of seizures but not others. Occasionally, some complementary treatments may actually make certain kinds of seizures worse. It is important that you know what kind of seizure you (or the person on whose behalf you are reading this book) experience. We have used the current terminology recommended by the ILAE to describe different seizure types throughout this book, i.e. 'seizures without impaired awareness', 'focal seizures with impaired awareness', 'generalized seizures', and 'status epilepticus'. However, people with epilepsy often have their own descriptions for their particular seizures, names which are clear and concise and which clearly delineate them from other events and which may date from the era in which they were first diagnosed.

Why you must continue to take your drugs

At the outset, it is important to stress that all of the treatments discussed in this book have been evaluated as 'add-on' therapies. That is, they have been used in addition to anti-epileptic drugs. If you are taking anti-epileptic drugs, it is extremely important that you continue to take them. Sudden discontinuation of these medications can have a devastating effect on seizure control and can, on occasion, lead to status epilepticus or even death. Any reduction in anti-epileptic medications should be made very gradually, under close medical supervision. This holds true, even if you think you have discovered a possible 'miracle cure'.

2

The importance of evidence

Nowadays, new drug treatments have to undergo rigorous tests before they can be offered to people. Doctors not only have to be sure that the treatments they offer will not harm their patient before they can proceed, they also have to have very good reasons to think the treatments they offer will help the person. Once a treatment has been proven to be safe and effective, there are strict controls in place to ensure that the drugs manufactured meet rigorous quality standards. In real life, finding the best treatment for every individual can be a hit-and-miss affair but, nevertheless, these principles guide every treatment offered.

With regards to harm, all medications undergo extensive safety tests before they are allowed to be prescribed. Often they have been taken by healthy people before they are tested in people with the illness they are designed to treat. It is the results of these tests, called clinical trials, that give doctors the reason to think that a new treatment may help their patients. These trials have to be conducted very carefully to ensure that the evidence upon which the doctor is going to base the decision to treat his or her patient is sound.

A fair test

'Before and after' measurements are an integral part of a fair test to see if a treatment has worked. However, a truly fair test is a far more complicated affair. A double-blind, randomized, placebo-controlled trial is currently one of the best tests available to see whether a new treatment works. This sounds like complicated medical jargon, but each part of the phrase actually describes a key part of the fair test. A 'placebo-controlled' trial means that not everyone in the study gets the new treatment. Usually, half of the participants get the treatment and the other half get a placebo, something that resembles the real treatment but has the important part missing. In trials of new medications, the participants in the placebo half of the study may get a pill that looks like the new medication, but actually just contains starch or sugar. In studies of other kinds of treatment it is often difficult for researchers to come up with a convincing placebo but, nevertheless, a fair test should involve a comparison group who are similar to the people who receive the treatment at the beginning of the trial. 'Randomized' means that the people who agree to take part in the study are randomly assigned to receive either the treatment or the placebo. This decision should not be based on how bad the person's symptoms are at the beginning, otherwise you could end up with an excess of people with the worst symptoms in the treatment group. This would not be a fair test. A truly random allocation takes any human bias out of the decision. 'Double blind' means that neither the doctor nor the participant in the trial knows whether they are receiving the real treatment or the placebo. They only find out once the study has finished. While this is relatively easy to achieve when testing pills (using third parties to dispense the medication and intricate codes), it is more difficult to 'blind' the participants and therapists when testing alternative treatments.

It is impossible to use these experimental designs in the study of some treatments, such as pet therapy, where it is fairly obvious whether someone has been allocated a dog or not! Nevertheless, fair tests can be still be devised with before and after measurements and comparisons with other people in a similar position who have not adopted a dog or a cat. (See Chapter 18 for other ways that have been devised to test whether pets can be helpful for people with epilepsy.) So, while a double-blind, randomized, placebo-controlled trial is one of the best methods we can use to see whether a new treatment really is effective, studies that fulfil all these criteria are quite rare. Nevertheless, it is a useful yardstick against which to measure the quality of evidence for *any* intervention, medical or otherwise, since the basic framework of the controlled trial is a fair test for all treatments that purport to have a beneficial effect on seizures.

The importance of large group tests

Why do we need to test new treatments on large groups of people? If five people try a new treatment and four get better, cannot we just extrapolate this information to say that 80 per cent of people will get better on the new treatment? Unfortunately, not. There may be many reasons (completely unrelated to the new treatment) why the four people could have got better. These individual variations get washed out in large groups where the real effect of the treatment being investigated can shine through all the background clutter. This is why anecdotal reports of 'miracle cures' based on a single person's experiences are not very useful to the wider epilepsy community. There may be many reasons why an individual's seizure control has improved, including natural fluctuations of the disease. These individual peaks and troughs in seizure control can be misattributed to all sorts of completely coincidental irrelevant factors, including, in some cases, the apparent cure. It is also not clear from some case studies whether or not the individual actually had epilepsy to begin with. For example, non-epileptic attack disorder can look very similar to epilepsy (as the name suggests), but the treatments are very different. Unless one is sure that the person had epilepsy to begin with, one cannot be sure that the apparent cure will work for epilepsy. Although the value of single case studies may be limited when it comes to being sure that a treatment approach really works, they can give us vital information when it comes to dangerous side effects of some medications and therapeutic approaches.

Collecting your own evidence

Many people will be given a seizure diary by their doctor when they are first diagnosed with epilepsy. These booklets are designed to help someone with epilepsy record when and where their seizures occur. They provide valuable data for the doctors to help them see whether the treatments they have offered are working. Seizure diaries are also one of the best tools someone with epilepsy has at their disposal to help them get to know their own epilepsy. Using a diary, you may notice that your seizures are more likely to occur at particular times of the day, week or month. Diaries kept over many years can help to identify seasonal variations in the frequency of seizures (see Chapter 14). The more you know about your epilepsy, the better you will be able to design your own 'fair test' to see if any new treatments you try really do work. If you find that you are less likely to have seizures in the summer for example, it would be important to bear this in mind if you introduce a new treatment in May. It might look like the treatment is having a good effect, but in actual fact the number of seizures you have that summer may be the same as previous years, when you were not taking the new treatment. In this case, it would be important to take these seasonal variations into account and perhaps wait into the autumn and winter months before judging the effectiveness of the new complementary treatment in controlling your seizures.

Before you start a new treatment, it is worth taking some time to think about how the treatment might affect you. Having fewer seizures is the ultimate goal for most people, but some complementary treatments for epilepsy may help you in other ways. You may find that your seizures do not last as long, or that you recover more quickly afterwards. Other treatments may improve your mood and may be worthwhile pursuing in that respect, even if you do not notice any appreciable effect on the number of seizures you experience. The more alert you are to the wider changes that can happen after you start a new treatment, the better you will be able to judge whether or not it is worth pursuing. Seizure diaries have ample space for you to record all kinds of information that you may feel is relevant. E-diaries are also available on the internet and as mobile phone applications. Please see the Useful addresses section at the back of this book for information on how to get a seizure diary if you do not already have one.

The placebo effect

Medical trials of new treatments are often measured against placebos. As described earlier, a placebo is a dummy medication; something that looks like real medicine, but is actually a harmless substitute. But the strange thing about placebos is that they also seem to work as effective treatments for a wide variety of illnesses and conditions, ranging from gastric ulcers to depression, chronic pain to angina. The placebo effect can also be seen in studies of epileptic seizures.

A study from Germany in 2011 found that over 80 per cent of doctors admitted to prescribing placebos for their patients; treatments that they had no reason to think would work. Many of these patients reported an improvement in their symptoms following the apparent treatment. The more expensive and complex a placebo treatment is, either in terms of its monetary value, or in the time and effort it requires from the recipient and medical staff, the more effective it appears to be. So, more people respond to an injection of harmless saline (salt water) than those taking sugar tablets. In turn, those taking many tablets are more likely to respond than those taking just one a day. Even the colour of a placebo tablet has been shown to affect how people respond to it.

In studies that have been designed to see if new treatments work for epilepsy, researchers often compare 'responder rates'. A responder rate is the percentage of people in a trial who respond to a new treatment; that is, get better. Researchers normally decide what would constitute a real improvement in the condition before they start the study. This stops any bias creeping in when they come to analyse the results. In studies of new treatments for epilepsy, the bar is normally set at 50 per cent. That means that a person has to have a reduction in seizures of at least 50 per cent when they are taking the new treatment for it to be judged effective, and for the person to be deemed a 'responder'. The higher the percentage of responders (or the responder rate) in a trial of a new treatment, the more effective it is. Responder rates are also normally reported for people who received the placebo treatment, and/or no new treatments at all, for comparison purposes to help doctors work out just how effective the new treatment is.

In epilepsy trials, the responder rate for placebo treatments is around 12 per cent. This means that more than one in ten people receiving a placebo treatment to control their seizures may get a reduction of 50 per cent of more in the number of seizures that they experience while they are undergoing the treatment. The responder rate in children receiving placebo treatments for epilepsy is even higher, approaching one in five. Generally, the response rates tail off as the time goes on, and seizure frequencies gradually return to their normal levels.

Even if it is not a permanent cure, the placebo effect in treating epilepsy is still a powerful force and should not be underestimated. So how does it work?

The placebo effect is not fully understood by doctors, but there are three possible components. Some people think that the apparent effects of the placebo treatment are just natural variations in the course of someone's epilepsy that have been misattributed to an irrelevant event. People may be more likely to seek out a new treatment when their seizures are at their worst. Unless an increased number of seizures is reflecting a serious deterioration in someone's underlying medical condition (rare), it is likely that the rate of their seizures would return to a more normal level over time, regardless of what treatment is offered. Doctors call this return to normality after a bad spell 'regression to the mean' and many think that it explains at least part of the placebo effect in trials of new epilepsy treatments.

The Hawthorne effect

Others think that part of the response seen in placebo treatment may be due to something psychologists call 'the Hawthorne effect'. The productivity of workers in the Hawthorne Works, a factory complex outside Chicago, was studied extensively by psychologists during the 1920s. The experimenters found almost all of the changes that they made to the workers' environment resulted in a *temporary* increase in production. The production rates would gradually return to normal over the following weeks. Some psychologists argue that the increased production rates were due to the workers responding to the interest shown in them by the team conducting the studies. They argue that similar things may be happening when someone is enrolled on a medical trial and receives lots of input and attention from the medical team as a result. But this can only be a partial explanation for the placebo effect in epilepsy, as it is not clear how lots of medical attention and a desire to please the study team would result in a noticeable change in seizure frequency, however strong the will of the researchers and the participants.

The remarkable power of the placebo effect is illustrated neatly by an American study published in 2010 that reported an astonishing placebo effect in dogs with epilepsy. Nearly 80 per cent of dogs in a placebo-controlled trial of canine anti-epileptic medications experienced a decrease in seizures after they had started to take the empty pills. Thirty per cent of the dogs could be considered 'responders' in the traditional sense, in that they had a reduction of greater than 50 per cent in the number of seizures they experienced. How could this be? It is unlikely that the trip to the vet engendered any feelings of warmth or being cared for in the dogs since, on the whole, few dogs enjoy veterinary encounters or appear to show any awareness that these visits may be beneficial so, in this instance, the Hawthorne effect almost certainly was not at play. Genuine regression to the mean in their underlying conditions may explain some of the improvements in some of the dogs, but was unlikely to be responsible for the improvements on the scale seen in the study. These findings are quite baffling until one realizes that it was the 'all too human' owners that were responsible for monitoring the seizure frequencies in their pets, before and after treatment. This study appears to prove that the unconscious placebo effect is so powerful in people, it even works by proxy.

Trying something new

Although we are not clear how it works, it is clear that trying something new may have at least a temporary effect on seizure control for those where new medications are not an option, and where existing medications have failed to completely control seizures. If it is a placebo effect, the improvement may wear off over a few months. A real therapeutic effect would be expected to last longer. Try not to be disheartened if some of the new treatments you may try do not lead to lasting results. It is unlikely (although not impossible) that any of the treatments described in the subsequent chapters will prove a miracle cure for your seizures. But it is possible that by cycling though a number of different treatment regimes and strategies over the course of a year you may be able to use the placebo effect to your advantage.

3

Stress

The human body is an extremely complex system. Many of the alternative therapies discussed in this book are designed to help you achieve balance and harmony within this system. Different therapeutic traditions invoke a variety of ideas to represent this balance: for example, 'yin' and 'yang' in Chinese medicine (see Chapter 9), the basic elements in Ayurvedic traditions (Chapter 8), and the rhythms manipulated in cranial sacral therapy (Chapter 12). Many of these approaches include a spiritual element. The underlying idea is the same; balance is the ideal that one should strive for.

Stress refers to anything that puts a system under pressure and disturbs its natural equilibrium. In the case of the human body, this stress can take many forms. It may come from external factors as the body struggles to adjust, for instance, to excessive noise, light or pollution. The human body can also be stressed on a physiological level by poor nutrition or drugs that are introduced into the system.

The form of stress that we are most familiar with on a day-to-day basis is the psychological kind. This is the type of stress that stems from our worries and anxieties that we cannot cope. These various forms of stress often merge into each other. Many people find their workplace stressful and feel exhausted after a day's work. Harsh lighting, difficult colleagues and looming deadlines with no time for lunch mean that the body will have been subjected to a wide range of stressors by the end of the working day. Knowing that it all starts again in a few hours on the following day does not help either. Very high levels of stress can also be induced by life events over which we have little control, for example illness and death in people we are close to, or natural disasters. For some people, just watching television reports of devastating events happening thousands of miles away, such as the 2011 Japanese tsunami and its aftermath, can increase their levels of stress.

Feelings of stress represent part of the human body's response to a perceived threat or danger. As soon as we become aware of a threat, or sometimes just the increased possibility of danger, our body reacts by releasing hormones such as cortisol and adrenaline, getting us ready for action. These chemicals make us more alert and physically prepare our muscles so that we are ready to either fight or run away fast from the danger. This is called the 'flight or fight response'.

Far back in our evolutionary history, almost all the threats we faced were to life and limb. However, the very same system kicks in today when the boss shouts at you, or your bus is caught in traffic when you are already late for an appointment. The hormones that prepare us to run away or fight are still released, but neither situation requires a physical response. This leaves the body in an unbalanced, uncomfortable state. If the increased levels of adrenaline and other chemicals the body produces in response to a perceived threat are not used to fuel a physical reaction, the high levels of these hormones coursing through the body can start to cause physical damage. Most people are aware that perpetually high levels of stress play a significant part in the development of heart disease. Scientists have now also found that high levels of cortisol, a key hormone released by the body during times of stress, can also affect the brain. Post-traumatic stress disorder (PTSD) is a neuropsychiatric condition that affects people who have been through a very traumatic event. They can be troubled by vivid flashbacks of the incident for many years. They also have elevated levels of cortisol in their blood, for months and sometimes years after the event. It is as if the body has been unable to reset itself back to normal levels and it keeps the individual in a perpetual state of readiness to confront danger. MRI studies have shown that, over time, these high levels of cortisol begin to damage parts of the brain, particularly the hippocampi, brain structures that are often involved in epilepsy.

Stress is not all bad. A certain amount of stress can help you in some situations. It is difficult to really concentrate properly if you are feeling too relaxed. This is why 'exam nerves' can help students, making them more mentally alert on their big day.

Too much stress

However, too much stress can push someone over the edge, and make them far less effective than they could be. It is almost impossible to concentrate properly if you are under too much stress. Psychologists use a rainbow-shaped curve on a graph to describe the effects of stress on performance. Initially, as the stress increases so does performance, but as stress levels continue to rise, performance goes downhill.

It is not a good idea to eliminate stress entirely from our lives. At the right level, stress hormones can make us feel excited, even exhilarated. This is why young children just cannot seem to keep still when they are excited. Their bodies react physically to the increased energy released by the stress hormones. As adults, we learn to suppress this natural physical response. Christmas, holidays and weddings are all associated with an increase in stress hormones, but we usually experience the changes within our bodies in response to these events as anticipatory excitement (for the most part at least – although it is easy to tip into feelings of rising panic, even on these happy occasions). The key to stress management is getting the balance just right.

Stress and epilepsy

Stress has close associations with seizures. From a chemical perspective, there is much evidence that suggests that stress hormones contribute to the pathology of epilepsy by lowering seizure thresholds, making a seizure more likely to occur.

There is also an abundance of clinical evidence linking stress to seizures. Although the story is more complex for people who develop epilepsy in childhood, many adults experience their first seizure in the context of a stressful event or series of events.

Jane

Jane's story illustrates this well. Jane was a student nurse in her early twenties who was fit and well with no history of epilepsy in her family. On New Year's Day her grandmother died, after a long illness. Just five days later, on the eve of the funeral, her grandfather also collapsed. He died a few hours later in hospital. On hearing the news, Jane's father, who had a history of heart disease, had a heart attack and was rushed into intensive care. That evening, Jane experienced the first of two generalized convulsions. While this series of calamitous events is certainly extreme, the timing is also important in this story. Christmas time and New Year often involve changes in routine and increased amounts of food and alcohol. It is likely that Jane's body was under an increased amount of physical stress due to these celebrations, even before her loved ones died and became ill. It was probably the cumulative effect of both the physical and psychological stresses in this difficult week that breached Jane's seizure threshold. Over 20 years later, Jane has not experienced any further seizures.

The physical state of the body has a significant impact on its seizure threshold. In very young children (under the age of five), seizures can occur if they develop a high temperature. These are called 'febrile convulsions' and do not always lead to epilepsy, in fact the majority do not. In May and June every year there is a peak in the number of young people turning up in the A&E departments of hospitals, up and down the country, having had their first seizure. Many are students who have stayed up all night and drunk to excess to celebrate the end of their exams. One report in the medical literature documents a series of brides who experienced their first seizures just prior to, or on, their wedding day. It is not just first seizures that are more likely to occur when someone is stressed. Once seizures have become established and someone has a diagnosis of epilepsy, they may begin to notice a pattern where their seizures are more likely to occur when they feel under pressure or are sleep deprived. This relationship is not always a perfect one-to-one correlation, probably because stress is just one of many factors that determine whether a seizure threshold is breeched. Nevertheless, the relationship is often there if you know what to look for.

Managing stress

There is much we can do to reduce the physical stresses on our bodies. Maintaining a healthy lifestyle with a good balanced diet has become the modern-day mantra to help us avoid cancer and heart disease. The fact is, a fit, healthy body is an advantage in almost every illness, including neurological conditions. Researchers in Sweden have recently found that people who are overweight in middle age increase their risk of developing Alzheimer's disease by 70 per cent. In epilepsy, as in life, the physically healthier you are, the better (see Chapters 5 and 6).

Managing psychological stresses may be more complex. A number of studies have looked at whether teaching formal relaxation methods to people with epilepsy results in better seizure control. Unfortunately, the results have not been very encouraging. While the participants in these studies generally felt less anxious, this did not translate into significantly fewer seizures in the group as a whole. One of the reasons why these treatment attempts have not been very successful may have been that they have employed a 'one size fits all' approach to stress management.

It is our reaction to a stressor that determines whether or not we become stressed by it. We are all very different in what we find stressful on a day-to-day basis. Some people seem to be able to shrug off minor arguments while others let the hurt fester for days. Some people daydream their way through a slow-moving queue, while others become increasingly irate as every minute ticks by. Individual differences in the ways in which we respond to these potentially stressful situations are due to a unique mix of our basic personality traits and things we have learnt along the way. Learning effective stress management will therefore be a very individual process: an appreciation that it is your personal reaction to an event that causes stress, not the event itself that is intrinsically stressful. This is the first step along the way. Finding new ways to respond to events you naturally perceive as stressful can be difficult. Sometimes, it involves undoing a lifetime of learning. Many of the techniques and therapies discussed in this book touch upon this to a greater or lesser degree. Some, such as the meditative techniques, explicitly teach relaxation. Others, such as homoeopathic medicine (Chapter 13) may work to reduce anxieties in a more oblique way (see also the section on the power of the placebo – Chapter 2). Finding a therapeutic approach that you believe in, and feel comfortable with, may go a long way to reducing the anxieties you may have about your epilepsy and the stress in your life generally. Regardless of the shaky scientific foundations of any approach, a reduction in stress that comes along with the therapy may make it a valuable weapon in your armoury against seizures.

4

Behavioural approaches to seizure control

For many people with epilepsy, it is the unpredictable nature of their seizures that makes the condition so difficult to live with. Approximately one in 20 people may have a very specific 'trigger' that sets off their seizure. These are called 'reflex epilepsies', and the most common is 'photosensitive epilepsy' where seizures are triggered by flashing lights. It is probably a reflection of the dramatic pairing of flashing lights and seizures that makes this rare epileptic phenomenon so well known among the general public. There can be few other medical conditions where the general public know so little about the most common features, such as focal seizures, yet instantly recognize a rare manifestation. Although the vast majority of people with epilepsy are completely unaffected by flashing lights, many signs and warnings on video games, rides, or anywhere where you may encounter strobe lighting will still warn of the dangers to all people with epilepsy.

More triggers

Although photosensitive epilepsy is the most common reflex epilepsy, there are many other types. In some people, seizures are triggered by visual patterns, such as moving escalator steps or bold stripy patterns that are in sharp contrast to the background. This means that their seizures may be triggered by bright, geometric wallpaper prints, or even clothing. Seizures can also be induced in some people when they play certain video games or watch television. In 1997, an episode of *Pokemon* was reported to trigger seizures in 685 Japanese children and teenagers, most of whom had no previous history of epilepsy. Subsequent analyses of the programme suggested that it may have been the rapid alternation of deep-red and bright-blue flashes in the TV cartoon that triggered the seizures. These children would have had a predisposition towards photosensitive epilepsy, but had never been exposed to the right stimulus until they watched the TV cartoon. As a result of this incident, the regulations for technical aspects of television programming were tightened up to prevent any similar events in the future. This has not stopped a number of people since trying to recreate the effect with home-made videos posted on YouTube. These efforts are typically entitled 'Test for epilepsy' or similar, and while most fail to recreate an epileptogenic flickering effect at the right frequency to induce a photosensitive seizure, some do manage it. While many people appear to grow out of photosensitivity, it is recommended that children do not watch these videos on the internet.

It is not just visual patterns and flashes that can cause seizures. Seizures can also be triggered by specific patterns of thought. Mental arithmetic, making decisions and playing chess can all trigger seizures in some people with reflex epilepsy. Mahjong is a very popular strategic game in China that has its own reflex epilepsy associated with it. Seizures can also be triggered by reading. Seizures induced by argumentative talking and writing have also been reported as rare, reflex epilepsies. In addition to sight and thought processes, specific sensations have been reported to trigger reflex seizures in some people. There is even a case report in the medical literature of seizures triggered by a woman brushing her teeth. Numerous members of an extended family in India have 'hot water epilepsy' – seizures brought on by contact with hot water. There is a clear genetic component to this kind of epilepsy which has been passed down through a number of generations.

While people with reflex epilepsies can try to avoid known triggers for their seizures, it is not generally possible to predict exactly when a seizure will occur for the overwhelming majority of people with epilepsy. For some, seizures may be more likely in some circumstances than others. Some people find that they are more likely to have a seizure if they have not had enough sleep, or if they have drunk a lot of alcohol the previous day. Some women notice that their seizures tend to cluster around the time of their menstrual periods. A seizure may be more likely to occur if you are very anxious or if you find yourself in a particularly stressful situation. Although there may be an increased risk of a seizure in these circumstances, it is still impossible for most people with epilepsy to predict exactly when their seizures will happen. However, the comprehensive neurobehavioural approach challenges this assumption and argues that people with epilepsy may be able to develop much more control over their seizures than they think.

The comprehensive neurobehavioural approach to seizure control in epilepsy

Donna Andrews

The comprehensive neurobehavioural approach to seizure control in epilepsy was developed by a young American woman called Donna Andrews. She developed epilepsy at the age of 18 following encephalitis. Having had a very bad experience with anti-epileptic medications, she devised a system of very careful observation and recording of her seizures, and the events that preceded each one, and worked on ways of 'diverting' a seizure before it fully developed. Eventually, she found that she could completely control her seizures. She teamed up with a neurologist who was interested in neurofeedback [see Chapter 16] and together they created the Andrews/Reiter comprehensive neurobehavioural treatment programme.

This programme is based on the belief that most seizures do not begin suddenly or inexplicably, despite this being the perception of many people with epilepsy. Identifying common factors that lead to the onset of seizures is critical in the Andrews/Reiter (AR) treatment programme. Although triggers in reflex epilepsies are fairly straightforward and simple, the AR approach argues that triggers for other kinds of seizures may also exist: they are just multiple and interactive, dependent upon the region of the brain involved. Triggers can be physical (disturbed sleep, missed medication), external (people, places and situations), or internal (emotional reactions, anxiety or stress). The AR approach suggests that seizures originating in the right hemisphere of the brain may be triggered by fear, guilt or sadness, while anger, frustration and excitement may trigger seizure activity in the left hemisphere. In the AR approach all aspects of seizure history are carefully documented, including where the seizure occurred, what was happening both immediately and days, even months, beforehand. Sleep patterns, work and social changes, dietary habits and emotional states are also carefully documented in order to build up a picture of the fullest possible context in which the seizure occurred. For example, it would not be sufficient to just record that a seizure occurred at work in the morning; but rather, you would need to note down exactly what you were doing, who was there with you, how you were feeling, what you were thinking about, what you were about to do etc., when the seizure occurred. The ultimate goal of these very detailed analyses is to discover dependable warnings for seizures and to become aware of the triggering mechanism for your own epilepsy. In addition to managing their triggers, participants on the programme are also trained to use deep breathing techniques to try to abort a seizure, when one does occur, before they lose awareness. Deep diaphragmatic breathing is a technique employed in many relaxation techniques and involves deep, controlled breaths from the diaphragm. People are encouraged to take a diaphragmatic breath as soon as they feel that they are beginning to depart from their normal state.

What's the evidence?

This approach has not been evaluated with a randomized control trial, but the results from 11 controlled case studies have been published. Their stories are very different.

26-year-old computer programmer

A 26-year-old man had a fear of measuring up to the standard he had set for himself. He worked as a computer programmer but often took a longer than his colleagues to complete tasks, and his boss thought he was slow. This pressure at work was deemed to be a significant stressor in his life, and following sessions with a comprehensive neurobehavioural therapist he recognized the effect his job was having on him. He found a new job, with less pressure, and also enrolled on a part-time course in computer engineering which boosted his self-esteem. At the start of the programme, he was experiencing five seizures a month. One year later, his seizures were completely controlled by medication.

Nine-year-old girl

In another case, therapy revealed that a nine-year-old girl, who had had epilepsy since the age of four, felt hurt and angry when people did not listen to her. She was worried by thoughts that bad things were about to happen and was sure that something evil lived in the woods behind her house. She was very angry that her parents did not believe her. The solution to reducing her anger and anxiety involved teaching her parents to listen to her concerns and take them seriously. One year later, the girl's seizures had reduced from eight a year to zero, and she had also come off all her anti-epileptic medication.

As case series go, these are relatively well controlled studies. The diagnosis of epilepsy was confirmed by a neurologist for all the participants and proper measurements of seizure frequency were taken before and after the treatment. However, while these case studies may offer some hope to people whose medications do not completely control their medication, it is very important to remember the limitations of this kind of evidence. Although these stories are encouraging and suggest that this approach may work for some people, they do not give us any idea of what proportion of people with epilepsy may respond to these methods. These positive responses to the therapy may be very rare. Proper randomized, controlled trials to assess whether this really is a viable treatment option for people with epilepsy still need to be done.

Will it work for you?

Getting to know your epilepsy has an intuitive appeal. Many people know that their seizures are more likely to happen at some times than others. The very detailed analyses that the comprehensive neurobehavioural approach involves may help to hone this knowledge further. Just keeping a more detailed record in your seizure diary may help you identify a possible trigger that you may not have been aware of previously. This approach may be particularly useful for people with rare seizures. However, for many people with epilepsy, their seizures are just too frequent, or the triggers may be too complex and too far integrated into their everyday lives, to enable them to be clearly disentangled. It is not always easy or practical to control the level of stress in our lives. We may all aspire to get a dream job, where we feel valued and fulfilled, but most of us are stuck with what we can get. The options for reducing stress are also limited if your primary source of stress comes from living with a teenager (or two!)

Developing an awareness of pre-seizure changes may also be challenging for some. Although some people may experience warning sensations prior to a seizure, seizures appear to come out of the blue for others, giving them no chance to make themselves safe or signal to their friends what is happening. Most people are amnesic for the events that occur during a seizure, and it can also be difficult to reconstruct a clear picture of exactly what was happening immediately beforehand also. This makes it difficult to subsequently recognize any immediate pre-seizure changes when they occur again.

The diaphragmatic breathing technique used in the comprehensive neurobehavioural approach has been proven to reduce anxiety and is an integral part of many relaxation techniques. It is relatively easy to master and can be implemented anywhere. While it reduces anxiety, it may not be effective in aborting seizures for everyone and the results are likely to vary with the individual, and the nature of their epilepsy. Indeed, some people may be better able to abort seizures by increasing their alertness, rather than relaxing. If you can identify pre-seizure changes (that give you a small window of opportunity to try to abort an impending seizure), you may be able to experiment with different techniques, if diaphragmatic breathing doesn't work for you.

In practical terms, it may be difficult for you to instigate the complete comprehensive neurobehavioural approach alone. There is a relatively inexpensive handbook available that will guide you though the basic steps (see the Useful addresses section at the back of this book for more details). However, remember that some therapeutic input from a psychologist was also available to the people who have been presented as success stories in the medical literature. This undoubtedly helped them to gain a clear understanding of wider aspects of their lives that they were dissatisfied with, and led to many of them making life-changing decisions such as changing jobs, embarking on a new career and even instigating divorce. Many psychologists in the UK may be unfamiliar with the comprehensive neurobehavioural approach in epilepsy. If you do wish to engage a psychologist to help you formulate ideas about possible triggers (and their solutions), it may be helpful to pass on the original scientific paper (see Useful addresses) to your chosen therapist so they know how to help structure their sessions with you.

In summary, the comprehensive neurobehavioural approach to seizure control has an intuitive appeal. Although its aims are ambitious and it is likely that only a few will be able to achieve the complete seizure control gained by its originator, the diary methods may help you gain a better understanding of your epilepsy and possible triggers for your seizures. Unlike many of the approaches discussed later in this book, there are no known side effects to this approach. And that, as you will learn if you read on, is a huge plus.

5

Exercise

People who exercise regularly live longer, are less likely to develop heart disease and cancer, and are less depressed than people who live sedentary lifestyles, i.e. those who rarely, if ever, move quickly under their own steam. Exercise is good for us. Aerobic exercise is particularly good for us. Any physical activity that gets our heart beating faster makes us fitter. The more often this is repeated, the fitter we get, and the fitter our bodies are, the better equipped we are to fight almost every disease or ailment we ever encounter. This is not to say fit people do not get ill. Of course they do, but on the whole they are significantly less likely to develop some of the most serious health problems, and even when they do develop them, they tend to survive for longer. This makes sense. Our bodies work best when the amount of fat we have is in the correct proportion to our lean tissue (muscle tissue without fat), and our heart and lungs are strong and able to supply and deliver the oxygen we need throughout our body. Although your brain is only about 2 per cent of your body mass, it uses up approximately 20 per cent of your oxygen consumption every day. It needs the right fuel to function effectively. This is influenced to some extent by diet (see Chapter 6), but the delivery system also has to be effective. To view brain function as separate from other vital organs when it comes to fitness is a mistake. Obesity is not only associated with an increased risk of developing dementia in old age, but it is also associated with increased cognitive impairments in middle age. Brain health and function is closely linked to physical condition. It follows that exercise and physical fitness may have an effect on seizure thresholds.

Epilepsy and exercise

For many years, scientists thought that physical exercise might actually trigger seizures in people with epilepsy. Although the physical fitness that comes from exercise is undoubtedly a good thing, exercise itself is also a form of stress and stress is a significant trigger for many people with epilepsy (see Chapter 3). In order to test this idea, Brazilian scientists studied two groups of rats, both of whom had a genetic mutation that meant they would have seizures. They put one group to work out daily on a rat treadmill, just like a miniature version of the running machines you would find in a gym, and left the other group to wander around their cage. The researchers were fully expecting the exercising rats to have more seizures but that is not what they found. It was the rats who did not exercise who had significantly more seizures than the ones who had been on the treadmill every day. Although the body may be stressed by exercise, studies in humans suggest that this kind of stress may have beneficial effects on brain function. During exercise, the brain receives messages from all over the body. This may inhibit seizures. The endorphins released during exercise may also act as a natural anticonvulsant.

One study of people with epilepsy found that the abnormal brainwaves recorded on their electroencephalograms (EEGs) disappeared when they walked with heavy packs on their backs or did knee bend exercises. Another study found the same effect when monitoring the EEGs of people using an exercise bike. Hyperventilation (rapid, fast breathing) is one of the techniques used to elicit abnormal brain waves on the EEG during routine testing. However, it appears that hyperventilation during exercise actually improves the EEG for most people with epilepsy. This is probably because the rapid breathing brought on by exercise is part of the body's natural compensatory attempts to re-establish balance, whereas rapid breathing out of this context actually creates an imbalance.

Competitive sport can generate pressure

Most sports require the player to be alert and paying attention; you literally need to be 'on the ball' to succeed. A number of scientists have argued that the increased alertness associated with this kind of exercise is an important part of the mechanism that promotes fewer seizures in people with epilepsy. However, the competitive element of some sports can be also associated with a huge pressure to win. This pressure is particularly acute in team games where others are relying on you. There are a number of stories in the medical literature of people experiencing seizures during the crucial part of a match.

16-year-old boy

One 16-year-old boy was involved in a very tense basketball game. The two teams in the championship final had been extremely closely matched throughout the game, with the advantage changing sides many times. The boy had a seizure in the final minute of the game. Since he had trained hard all season and played in many previous matches without incident, it probably was not the physical exertion in this particular match that lead to this seizure, but the additional psychological tension and mounting excitement throughout the match associated with the desire to win that breached his seizure threshold.

A number of professional athletes with epilepsy have also reported that their seizures tend to occur before, during or after a competitive match, while they never seem to happen during training sessions, which are often more physically demanding than the matches themselves. While there are cases of people who clearly experience exercise-induced seizures purely triggered by physical activity, this is a very rare form of epilepsy.

Sudden unexpected death in epilepsy (SUDEP) is a rare but devastating phenomenon. We still have much to learn about the mechanisms that lead to sudden death, but some scientists have argued that regular physical exercise may protect people from SUDEP. These arguments are theoretical at present, and while they make sense, there is no clear clinical evidence to support this. However, there is clear evidence that exercise has a markedly positive impact on bone health, particularly on bone mineral density (BMD). Since the long-term use of many anti-epileptic drugs is associated with a loss of BMD over time, exercise is an excellent way of protecting and maintaining bone health in epilepsy, together with a healthy diet and vitamin D supplements (see Chapter 6).

Exercise and seizure control

Although there have been many studies looking at the effects of exercise in animals with epilepsy and on EEG waves in people, there are disappointingly few trials of exercise as an add-on treatment for seizures in people. One study looked at the effectiveness of twice-weekly, 60-minute sessions, involving aerobic dancing with strength training and stretching, over the course of 15 weeks. Seizure frequencies were recorded by the participants for three months before they began exercising, then during the exercise period and for three months after they stopped the classes. The researchers found that the number of seizures the participants reported reduced significantly over the weeks that they were exercising compared to the weeks before and after. Interestingly, the seizures returned when the exercise programme had finished. The researchers felt that 15 weeks was too short a time to establish the radical lifestyle change that incorporating regular exercise into everyday routines involves.

Other studies have not found a significant effect of exercise on seizure frequency but have recorded beneficial effects on measures of psychological and social well-being. It is likely that the lack of any significant effects on seizure control in some of these studies were due to the very small number of participants and relatively short periods of exercise studied. Exercise needs to be sustained over many months for real improvements in physical fitness to emerge. It seems probable that any improvements in seizure control associated with exercise will occur over a similar timeframe.

Will it work for you?

Unless you are unlucky enough to have exercise-induced seizures, it is likely that you will benefit from physical exercise if you have epilepsy. Although you are unlikely to become completely seizure-free if you instigate a moderate exercise programme, over time it may result in a noticeable decline in the number of seizures you experience. Improvements in mood and overall quality of life are also very likely to follow. Your bone health will increase and you may be protecting yourself from SUDEP. Exercise is also great way to deal with stress, which in turn may lead to a further reduction in seizures.

Your choice of exercise will be constrained to some extent by your epilepsy. Any sport where a seizure will result in severe injury or death is best avoided for obvious reasons. Examples include scuba diving, motor sports and many of the modern day extreme sports such as free climbing, parkour, snowboarding etc. Seizures that may occur while using various types of gym equipment (such as a treadmill) can also sometimes result in significant injuries if, for instance, body parts get trapped in the machinery. The best advice for choosing an activity is to imagine exactly what would happen if you had one of your habitual seizures in the middle of the exercise. Solo hang-gliding and deep-sea diving are sports that require a constantly high level of vigilance, not just for success, but for survival. Risks associated with other potentially dangerous activities such as water sports and swimming can be managed to some extent by ensuring the adequate vigilance of lifeguards and accompanying friends.

Competitive boxing, with its integral risks of head injury, is not recommended for anyone concerned with the preservation of brain function, regardless of whether or not they have epilepsy. The British Medical Association (BMA) continues to campaign for a total ban on the sport in the UK. Their opposition to boxing is based on the fact that it results in chronic brain damage that is sustained cumulatively over time. Often, boxers do not become aware of the damage for a number of years, but in later life the effect of the brain damage can become very apparent with accelerated ageing and increased risks of early dementia.

While competitive sports may increase unhelpful psychological aspects of stress if someone's desire to win becomes paramount, these activities have the advantage of widening someone's social network. Feeling part of a team can confer many beneficial effects on mood and general psychological well-being. People with epilepsy should not therefore avoid competitive sports, but should be aware that having too much invested in the outcome of a match or game may lower their seizure threshold. By gradually increasing the challenge of each competition, people with epilepsy can train to cope with the stress of competition in the same way that they train physically to meet the demands of the sport.

Fortunately, most forms of exercise do not raise any special concerns for people with epilepsy. Jogging, racquet sports, and group exercise and dance classes are all relatively low risk activities. If you are very unfit, and are self-conscious about exercising in a group environment, numerous fitness and dance packages for video game consoles are available. These programmes allow you to exercise in your own home, at your own pace and many chart your progress along the way. They may be a useful introduction to exercise for people who need to build up their confidence when it comes to working out the relationship between exercise and their seizures.

Consistency and commitment

If you are thinking of instigating a fitness regime as a complementary approach to controlling your seizures, it is important to remember that the results will not be instant. Consistency and commitment are the key. If you do not regularly exercise devise a realistic programme of activities that you can stick to. This is a significant lifestyle change, and radical plans are likely to fall quickly by the wayside. The amount of exercise you will need to do to improve your physical fitness will very much depend on your starting point. If you currently do nothing, aiming for the current UK government guidelines of 30 minutes a day of moderate exercise, such as brisk walking, will be a good starting point. If you are already active, the staff in most gyms will devise a bespoke fitness regime for you when you join. In some areas, local gym membership can be prescribed by your GP.

6

Diet

In 1826, a French writer, Jean Anthelme Brillat-Savarin, published a book called *La Physiologie du goût* (*The Physiology of Taste*). In it, he wrote, 'Dis-moi ce que tu manges, je te dirai ce que tu es', which roughly translates as 'Tell me what you eat and I will tell you what you are'. 'You are what you eat' remains a phrase in common use today. It is literally true. From the moment we emerge from the womb, our growth from newborn baby to adulthood is fuelled entirely from the food we eat and the liquid we drink. But, while the phrase can be taken literally, Brillat-Savarin did not mean this. He meant that the food we eat has a significant bearing on our state of mind and physical health. He was right.

A century later, the idea that nutrition and health were inextricably linked had taken such a hold that one meat-producing company used it in their newspaper advertising campaign. Their 1923 advert for beef boldly claimed that 'Ninety per cent of the diseases known to man are caused by cheap foodstuffs. You are what you eat. A message brought to the public's attention by the United Meet [sic] Markets.' This was obviously in the days before the Advertising Standards Authority (ASA) challenged unfounded claims (and schoolboy spelling mistakes). Nevertheless, the importance of diet and nutrition in the prevention of many serious diseases, including some of the biggest killers in the West such as heart disease, diabetes and cancer, has been increasingly recognized over the past century. The importance of getting the message across to children and young people to capitalize on the preventative value of a good diet has not been lost on successive UK governments. The five-a-day campaign, promoting the aim of eating five pieces of fruit and vegetables a day, is now taught as part of the national curriculum to primary school children across the UK. In the more recent Change for Life campaign (2008–11), the UK government spent over £75 million in a multimedia campaign to get the message across.

It is beyond the scope of this book to discuss the general health benefits of a balanced diet. Lots of advice about healthy eating and recommended guidelines for sugar and fat are available on the UK National Health Service website (see the Useful addresses section at the back of this book for further information). Many people are already aware of what constitutes a healthy diet; it is sticking to it that is the problem. However, you may not be aware that certain food types and some dietary regimes may make seizures more or less likely in some people with epilepsy. This chapter examines the evidence for some of these dietary treatments for epilepsy.

Nutrition and epilepsy

The brain needs to be supplied with a very specific mix of amino acids, vitamins, minerals and fats to function properly. While the body can produce some of these itself, many need to come directly from the diet on a regular basis, as they are not readily stored. Some specific metabolic disorders can cause seizures. Vitamin B6 deficiency is usually apparent very early in life and leads to recurrent seizures. Fortunately, taking vitamin B6 supplements addresses the balance and controls the seizures. The role of other vitamins and minerals is more complex. The impact of some mineral deficiencies on seizure thresholds appears to rely on the ratio of one compound to another in the diet. Others need to be present in the diet at just the right level. For example, too much or too little copper can exacerbate seizures. It would be very difficult to design a completely new diet from scratch to ensure the adequate amounts and ratios of all the vitamins, minerals and fats we need. Fortunately, others have converted all the data and equations into a list of the foodstuffs we need to include in our diet. (Sources of information on a healthy balanced diet can be found at the back of this book in the Useful addresses section.) Your GP will also be able to refer you to a dietician who will be able to help you construct an individual diet plan that fits in with your lifestyle.

Although there are anecdotal reports of very sugary foods, or foods high in additives, triggering seizures in some people (particularly children), these effects have not been systematically studied in epi-lepsy populations. High levels of refined sugar in the diet certainly have effects throughout the body and particularly on the brain. We experience a 'sugar rush' after eating sweets as the blood transports large amounts of glucose directly to the brain. In response, the brain releases serotonin, a neurotransmitter which makes us feel happy. These effects can be very marked in children, and many parents are all too aware of the post-birthday cake frenzy that frequently overtakes birthday celebrations when the children have consumed large quantities of icing. High levels of blood sugar also prompt the pancreas to release large amounts of insulin to soak up the glucose to store for later use. Not only does this lead to weight gain, but it rapidly deprives the brain of energy, leading to the post-chocolate lethargy many of us are familiar with. This in turn leads to a craving for more sugar and so the cycle continues. Too much refined sugar in the diet eventually leads to an increased likelihood of type II diabetes and a significantly increased risk of dementia and stroke in later life. It is clear that eating high levels of refined sugar over time has a detrimental effect on brain function. You may notice that it also has an impact on the pattern of your seizures. Even if there is no discernable pattern connecting your intake of refined sugar to an exacerbation of your seizures, there is clear evidence from these other health domains that it should be eaten in moderation.

Antioxidants

Free radicals are highly reactive molecules that are formed when oxygen interacts with certain molecules. Once formed, free radicals can trigger a domino effect, causing damage to cells over time. This damage will eventually result in the death of the cell. Free radicals are thought to play an important role in the ageing process. Antiox-idants are the body's natural defence against free radicals. Vitamins A, C and E are natural antioxidants and clinical studies have shown that sufficient intake of these vitamins over time can reduce the risk of certain cancers developing and slow down the progression of degenerative diseases such as Alzheimer's and Parkinson's disease.

There is also evidence from laboratory studies that seizure activity increases the levels of free radicals in the blood. Natural antioxidants can be used to compensate for these increases in people with epilepsy and, fortunately, this is easily done. In addition to the widely available vitamin supplements of A, C, and E, the vitamins can also be found in many foods that constitute a healthy diet, such as fruit (particularly citrus varieties), vegetables (sweet potatoes, carrots and spinach are excellent sources), and whole grain foods (cereals and wholegrain breads and pastas).

In addition to tackling the unwanted rise in free radicals associated with seizure activity, some antioxidants may also play a role in reducing seizures. In one placebo-controlled study of vitamin E, where neither the doctors nor the children taking part knew whether they were taking the vitamin or a placebo, vitamin E was associated with a significant reduction in seizure frequency. There was no change in the placebo group. Although the numbers in the trial were small (just 24 children took part), the results of this trial are encouraging. Unfortunately, a second trial looking at the effectiveness of vitamin E in a larger group of 43 people failed to replicate the success of the earlier study and the researchers found no differences between the placebo group and those taking the vitamin E.

The levels of vitamin E taken by the children in the smaller study (400 IU/day) were many times the recommended dietary allowance (RDA) for the age group, which is currently 10 IU–16 IU/day. RDAs are based on the average daily level of intake required to meet the nutrient requirements of the vast majority of healthy people. In addition to RDAs, there are also guidelines regarding the tolerable upper intake level for vitamins and minerals. The tolerable upper intake level for young children aged one to three years is 300 IU/day raising to 1,500 IU/day for adults. This is the maximum daily intake that is *unlikely* to cause adverse health effects. Intake above these levels may be associated with minor side effects such as stomach upset and diarrhoea. Very large amounts of vitamin E, hundreds of times greater than the daily recommended amount, may be associated with more serious side effects in some people, particularly if they are taken for long periods of time; an increase in the risk of stroke and haemorrhage has been reported in some studies. Excessive doses of vitamin E are unnecessary and may result in more harm than good. However, taking a vitamin E supplement that ensures that you have the recommended daily amount is unlikely to do you any harm and, as a bonus, you may notice improvements in your complexion as well as an improvement in your seizure control.

Minerals

The human body relies on 16 minerals to function properly. Many of us are familiar with the fact that we need calcium for bone health and iron to give us energy, but other minerals we may usually only associate with chemistry lessons (and the periodic table), such as zinc, copper and manganese, are also essential for health. A healthy diet will normally ensure that we get enough of these, but some studies have suggested that seizures can be associated with low levels of these essential minerals. One study analysed the hair of people with and without epilepsy. Hair strands grow slowly and contain a record of the levels of minerals available to the body over time. Levels of copper, magnesium and zinc were lower in people with epilepsy, compared to those who did not have seizures. Interestingly, this was the case even for the people who were not taking any anti-epileptic drugs. This suggests that there is something about having seizures that is associated with lower levels of the minerals in the body. Magnesium is needed to help the body absorb calcium and although there have been no randomized-controlled trials of magnesium supplements, two group studies have reported a reduction in seizures in people who have taken supplements. In the diet, magnesium is found in green vegetables, nuts, seeds and whole grains. Some anti-epileptic medications may also interfere with the absorption of zinc from foods. Foods high in zinc include lean meats, poultry, fish and offal, together with dairy products, eggs, whole grains, nuts and seeds.

Specialist diets

The idea of treating epilepsy via specialist diets is not new. Hippocrates described the case of a man whose seizures stopped when he fasted. Observations that complete fasting leads to a reduction in seizures were also made in early medical reports from the twentieth century. In one study reported in 1921, some participants were made to fast for up to 25 days. While their seizures may have diminished, it is unlikely that their quality of life improved significantly under such a draconian, unsustainable regime. It is probable that at least some of the effects of starvation on reducing seizures in these early studies were due to ketosis. Ketosis is a condition that occurs when the body starts to burn fat instead of glucose for energy. This can happen following starvation or a long physical training session when the body has run out of carbohydrates. After about 48 hours of this form of body stress, the brain starts to burn ketones, getting its energy directly from the fat stores, saving the glucose reserves for vital functions in an effort to avoid depletion of the protein store in the muscles. Ketosis, therefore, affects the way in which the brain functions and it appears to make seizures less likely for some people with epilepsy. While ketosis is always associated with starvation, it can also be induced with specialist diets. It is these diets that form the basis of dietary treatments for some children with epilepsy today.

The ketogenic diet

The classic ketogenic diet is extremely high in fat and very low in carbohydrates and proteins. Typically, over 90 per cent of energy comes from fat and only 10 per cent comes from protein and carbohydrates combined. Other variations include the medium chain triglyceride (MCT) ketogenic diet which has slightly more generous allowances for carbohydrate (15 per cent) and protein (10 per cent) but nevertheless maintains an extremely high fat content. This means that the diet will typically consist of cream, oils and butter, mayonnaise, eggs, some meat, limited vegetables and tiny amounts of fruit, bread, pasta and rice. The ketogenic diet has been studied extensively in children over the past ten years, not least because an influential Hollywood movie director, Jim Abrahams (famous for *Aircraft! Hot Shots!* and *Scary Movie 4*), made a film with Meryl Streep in 1997 based on the true story of his son's epilepsy. *First Do No Harm* tells the story of a boy so disabled by his seizures that his parents are forced to consider surgery. As he is about to go under the knife, they discover that the ketogenic diet may help him, and it does. He is saved from surgery and his seizures are controlled. The film did much to publicize the possibilities of the diet and a number of charitable organisations have been set up, both in the UK and the USA, to campaign for greater awareness of the treatment as a result.

Many studies have reported success in children who have very frequent seizures; however, there have only been two randomized controlled trials of the diet conducted to date. The first looked at the effects of the diet in children with very frequent seizures, occurring on a daily basis. In the group as a whole, the children who adhered to the diet experienced a 38 per cent decrease in seizure frequency. In the second trial, problems with the methodology of the study make the results more difficult to interpret, but the researchers did not find that the diet was particularly effective in reducing seizures.

Side effects of the ketogenic diet include vomiting, diarrhoea, constipation and hunger. Children have also been found to bruise more easily while on the diet. Renal stones may be more likely to form, particularly in children who are wheelchair-bound. Unsurprisingly, the diet is associated with raised blood cholesterol and growth can be impaired with long-term use. It can lead to a very restricted lifestyle, particularly in older children, and requires a very high level of supervision for success. There are some rare childhood epilepsy syndromes for which the ketogenic diet may be useful as an early treatment, including Doose Syndrome, Dravet Syndrome and West Syndrome. In all cases, the diet should be introduced under close medical supervision, normally on an inpatient basis in a hospital. A parent should never try to introduce the ketogenic diet without medical support and advice, and to do so would be dangerous for the child. There are some rare metabolic conditions where introduction of the ketogenic diet can trigger a potentially fatal metabolic crisis. Anybody considering the ketogenic diet therefore needs to be screened for these conditions before they change their dietary regime.

The majority of studies that have looked at the effectiveness of a ketogenic diet in controlling seizures have been in children. And the majority of the children who took part had very severe epilepsy, often in the context of an epilepsy syndrome. However, with the rise in popularity of the Atkins diet in the general population, which also induces ketosis, some studies have begun to look at the effectiveness of this diet in adults. As yet there have been no randomized-controlled trials in adults. Dangers of the ketogenic diet in adults include loss of bone density and menstrual irregularities in woman. The long-term effects of these diets on heart and vascular health in people with epilepsy are unknown, but legitimate concerns have been raised about the effects of the raised cholesterol level associated with such a high fat content in the diet.

Will it work for you?

For the majority of people with epilepsy, developing and maintaining a healthy, balanced diet will be the dietary intervention of choice. NHS guidelines are available online (see the Useful addresses at the back of this book) and if you require further guidance, your GP may be able to refer to you to a dietician. It is important to be aware of the distinction between a dietician and a nutritionist. 'Dietician' is a title protected by law in the UK. That means that anyone calling themselves a dietician must have completed formal training at degree level and must be registered with the UK Health Professions Council (HPC) in order to practise. Most dieticians practise within the NHS. 'Nutritionist' is not a protected title, which means that anyone can call themselves a nutritionist.

Specialist diet regimes may be useful for some children with specific epilepsy syndromes but should always be introduced under competent medical supervision, usually in an inpatient setting. These radical diets have been trialled less frequently in adults and may be associated with harmful long-term effects on bone and heart health.

7

Herbal remedies

The word 'herbal' tends to have benign connotations. 'Herbal' has become equated with 'natural' and 'gentle' in our society and advertisers use these strong associations to market everything from shampoo to sleeping pills. In fact, the label 'herbal' just means that a key ingredient of a medicine has been extracted from a plant. Although plants may be perceived as harmless, some of them contain powerful, even lethal, poisons. Others can cause skin irritations that can turn to burns if the skin is subsequently exposed to sunlight. Plants with these properties are not just found in exotic, remote jungles. There are probably some in your garden. Wistaria, daphne and delphinium are all poisonous if they are eaten. Other plants that may cause serious harm, even death, when eaten include digitalis, euphorbias, laburnum seeds and yew berries. Children are particularly vulnerable to these poisons. Some laurel leaves contain cyanide compounds, which can be released if hedge clippings are burnt in a bonfire. Most people grow up knowing that some mushrooms can be dangerous, even lethal, but few are aware of the plant poisons they may brush past every day. However, while some plants may be dangerous, many have remarkable medicinal qualities.

Man is not unique in recognizing the medicinal properties of plants. The study of self-medication in animals even has its own name, 'zoopharmocognosy': 'zoo' for animal, 'pharmo' for medicine, and 'cognosy' for knowing. From ants to elephants, animals make extensive use of the plants in their environment to treat their ailments. Many of the traditional remedies in folk medicine were developed following human observations of animal eating habits. The Navajo tribe in the USA acknowledge bears for their understanding of the antifungal, antibacterial and antiviral properties of the umbelliferae plant found in the south western corner of America.

In the Himalayas, the discovery that the roots of the Chota-chand plant contained an effective antidote for a potentially fatal snake-bite came from the observation that mongooses regularly sought and snacked on the plant before they started a fight with a cobra. One folklore tale of the discovery of coffee is even attributed to an Ethiopian shepherd, who noticed that his goats perked up considerably after they had eaten berries from wild coffee plants. Over one-fifth of the plants that chimpanzees habitually eat have little nutritional value but are effective medicines for stomach upsets and the treatment of parasitical infections.

Humans have long recognized the value of some plants in treating illnesses. The fact that primates appear to be able to pass on knowledge of useful plants from one generation to the next suggests that the relationship between plants and humans has a long history stretching way back into our evolutionary roots. Hippocrates, writing in approximately 400 BC, described the use of a powder made from the bark and leaves of a willow tree that was effective in relieving headaches, pains and fevers. Today, millions across the globe continue to use the very same active ingredient, salicylic acid, for the same symptoms. We now know it as aspirin. A fascinating review of the origins of modern medicines, published in 2001, identified 122 modern drugs in widespread use, obtained from 94 species of plants. The plants used to make 80 per cent of these drugs were also used to treat the identical or similar condition in one or many folk remedies from around the world. The authors of the review put forward some persuasive arguments for using plants, particularly those used in traditional medicines, as starting points for new drug developments.

While it may be foolhardy to ignore the wealth of ancient knowledge surrounding the medicinal use of plants, it is also true that many ancient cures were (and are) nothing of the sort. Unfortunately, this is particularly the case for herbal epilepsy treatments. This is partly because so many herbal treatments for epilepsy exist. Writing in 1850, Sir Edward Henry Sieveking, an eminent British neurologist, observed that, 'There is scarcely a substance in the world capable of passing through the gullet of a man that has not, at one time or another, enjoyed the reputation of being anti epileptic'.

It is difficult to find widely accepted guidelines for the herbal treatment of seizures, but the following are among the most frequently recommended for epilepsy today.

Bishopswort

Bishopswort is also known as betony, or wood betony. It is often marketed as a herbal remedy to induce calm and conquer anxiety. Although it does appear to reduce blood pressure, the cost may be diarrhoea, nausea and other gastrointestinal difficulties. There is no evidence that it is effective in controlling seizures.

Blue cohosh

Blue cohosh has many names and is marketed as blue ginseng, yellow ginseng, squawroot and papoose root. The seeds of the plant are bright blue. It has similar properties to those found in nicotine and it is used in herbal obstetric practice to induce labour, although there have been rare cases of heart failure in babies where blue cohosh was taken during the pregnancy. It is poisonous to children and should not be taken by adults with heart problems. Diarrhoea can be an adverse reaction. There is no evidence that it has any therapeutic effect in epilepsy.

Kava

Kava has many different names, the majority of which are a variation on the basic kava. Examples include kava-kava and ava. Like bishopswort, it is believed to have calming properties. However, while it may have a sedative effect, it can also induce high blood pressure, bloodshot eyes and diarrhoea. There is no evidence that it has any therapeutic effects in epilepsy. You may have noticed a theme developing here, both with the lack of any evidence that these herbal remedies work for epilepsy and the alarming regularity with which diarrhoea features as a frequent side effect. However, the side effects of kava-kava are not just limited to bowel discomfort. Liver transplants in 14 people have been linked to them taking kava-kava. Seven deaths have also been attributed to this herbal remedy.

Mistletoe

The 'kissing bough' you may hang over your door at Christmas is a highly toxic plant. Coma, cardiac arrest and psychosis (along with, you've guessed it, diarrhoea), are just some of the side effects associated with this plant. Unlike the other herbal remedies that have been discussed so far, mistletoe has been associated with seizures in clinical studies but, unfortunately, it tends to cause them rather than make them less likely.

Itchweed

The Harry Potter-esque itchweed is also known as American, false, green or swamp hellebore, or Indian poke. This plant has similar effects to some steroids and can be highly toxic, with effects on the heart, lungs and central nervous system. It should never be taken in pregnancy as it causes facial deformities during foetal development in the womb. In the context of all these negative effects, there is no evidence that it is effective in controlling seizures. In fact, seizures may occur if toxicity develops within the central nervous system, following the ingestion of itchweed.

Mugwort

Continuing in a Harry Potter-esque vein, mugwort is also sometimes marketed as an effective herbal treatment for epilepsy. It is a member of the daisy family, which sounds innocuous enough, but can cause contact dermatitis, allergic reactions and in extreme cases, anaphylaxis. It has no proven effects on seizures.

Ground holly

Nausea, vomiting and diarrhoea can be associated with ground holly, also known as pipsissewa or the rather more prosaic prince's pine or spotted wintergreen. There is no clinical evidence that it is effective at safe doses for epilepsy and it should not be consumed.

Skullcap

Skullcap, also known as helmet flower or hoodwort, is sometimes marketed as an anticonvulsant. It certainly seems to have some effects on brain function. Unfortunately, it is yet another herbal remedy that has been associated with causing seizures rather than curing them. Other problems associated with skullcap include confusion, stupor and cardiac arrhythmias.

Will it work for you?

Up until May 2011, it was legal to buy herbal remedies originating from any herbal medicine tradition over the counter. However, recognizing the potential dangers associated with some of these medicines, the EU brought in new legislation to govern access to these medicines. This came into force in the UK in May 2011. It is still possible to buy some herbal remedies over the counter if they have been registered with the UK Traditional Herbal Medicines Scheme. This scheme began in 2005 and all products registered are required to meet specific standards of safety and quality, with strict guidelines governing what can be mixed in with the product. This should reduce some of the dangers associated with adulteration in herbal medicine. Adulteration is the addition of dangerous substances into a herbal remedy, including arsenic, heavy metals and even pharmaceutical products. If a herbal medicine is registered with this scheme it will carry their green leaf logo on the packet.

The UK government has proposed that all herbal practitioners should be registered with the HPC in the future. However, this proposal has provoked fierce criticism from some doctors and scientists, who claim that regulating practitioners who offer unproven treatment methods will not offer the public any meaningful protection. Regardless of whether these proposed safeguards eventually come into force, these new regulations do not ensure that any herbal medications will be effective. For herbal medicines, the only burden of proof required is that they have been used 'traditionally' to treat whatever condition they are being prescribed for, for a minimum of 15 years. For herbal medicines, it seems that the longevity of an idea is adequate 'proof' that they work. Unfortunately, history tells us that the longevity of an idea does not really bear much relation to its accuracy. People believed that the world was flat for millennia, but it did not make it true. Any more than the very old idea, still around today in some parts of the world, that epilepsy is caused by demonic possession.

Although many of these herbal remedies have potentially powerful effects on body and brain chemistry, none have been proven to have clear anticonvulsant qualities in clinical trials. Many are associated with unpleasant, sometimes dangerous, side effects. Numerous herbal preparations may interact with anti-epileptic medications making them more or less potent. An increase in the potency of anti-epileptic medications may lead to toxicity; a decrease may result in a reduction in seizure control. This is the case even with some common herbal remedies that are not taken for epilepsy, such as ginko and evening primrose oil.

Although it is possible that one day the study of plant properties may lead to a breakthrough in seizure control, the evidence to date suggests that current herbal remedies are not effective treatments for epilepsy. If you are tempted to try a 'natural' remedy, remember that the distinction between many herbal tablets and prescription drugs may just be that the latter have been properly tested in clinical trials and that they continue to be fully regulated and controlled and cannot be prescribed for conditions in which they are not proven to work. If you are still tempted to try a herbal remedy, please tell whoever prescribes your anti-epileptic medications what you are taking and do not discount it as just 'herbal'. Your doctor will be able to advise you about any potential harmful interactions that are known about the remedy you wish to try and your own combination of anti-epileptic drugs.

8

Ayurvedic medicine

Ayu is Sanskrit for life, *veda* is Sanskrit for knowledge. The Vedas are a collection of ancient Indian texts. Indian tradition holds that the Vedas were revealed to wise men by Brahma, the Hindu god of creation, approximately 6000 BC. While they may not be 8000 years old, modern historians believe that the written records of ancient medical knowledge certainly date from before 1000 BC. The Ayurvedic system of medicine consists of three elements, or humours, within the human body: *vata* (air) *pitta* (bile) and *kapha* (phlegm). These basic elements are similar to the humours embraced thousands of years later in medieval European medicine. These elements were used in a broad sense by the ancient Hindus to understand human physiology. Imbalances between the elements are thought to be the source of illness and disease.

The Ayurvedic texts have much to say about epilepsy, covering symptoms, causes, diagnosis and treatment. They make the distinction between epileptic convulsions, pseudo seizures (attacks with a psychological origin), and apoplectic attacks (a loss of control associated with extreme anger). These alternative diagnoses for unexplained attacks (called 'differential diagnoses' in modern Western medicine) remain prominent in the minds of many modern epileptologists and neurologists today when they are faced with the conundrum of people who do not seem to respond to conventional treatments for seizures. The Ayurvedic texts also recognize four different types of epilepsy, all characterized by the sudden onset and equally sudden disappearance of symptoms. They document that most seizures spontaneously resolve without any treatment, but that one of the four forms of epilepsy is incurable. Again, these features of the condition are easily recognizable today in modern Western medicine.

However, in a significant departure from modern Western

approaches, in most Ayurvedic texts epilepsy is viewed as a psychiatric condition or a mental disease. Causes include immoral behaviour and gratuitous gratification. As the various humours become disturbed by this aberrant behaviour, the imbalance leads to build-ups and blockages, and eventually a seizure will occur.

Traditional Ayurvedic approaches to seizure first aid include blood-letting from the veins in the temples, and cauterisation of the parietal skull bones with needles. Avurvedic treatments for epilepsy begin with a purging of the system. This may involve the administration of a very strong emetic (a substance that will induce vomiting) and other purgatives to thoroughly clear out the digestive tract. Only when the person has been purged of all impurities do they move on to taking Ayurvedic medications. These medications are often mixed with other substances and cooked in ghee and other oils to make them more palatable. Some may be herbal; others involve elaborate preparations of animal products. One such complex animal-based prescription consists of fermented liquor made from wine sediment mixed with the dried and powdered, half-digested contents of a pig's stomach (the pig having been fed on boiled rice and the juice of a bhargi plant).

What's the evidence?

Advocates of Ayurvedic medicine point out that it is unwise to dismiss 4000 years of wisdom. While this deserves consideration, there are very few areas in our modern lives where we would share a common understanding with our ancestors who were living 400, never mind 4000, years ago. Subsequent scientific advances have made a nonsense of much of the rationale that underpins treatments that were developed even in the relatively recent past, including the late nineteenth and early twentieth centuries. See the chapters in this book on homoeopathy (Chapter 13) and manipulation therapies (Chapter 12) for prime examples. The idea that epilepsy stems from some kind of moral defect is common in many cultures and as recently as the 1940s the notion that people with epilepsy should not be allowed to have children in case they be mentally retarded was peddled in major Hollywood films: see *Dr Kildare's Crisis* (MGM Studios, 1940). When Ronald Reagan starred in a biopic of a famous baseball player who developed post traumatic epilepsy in *The Winning Team* (1952), the film studio forbade the scriptwriters to mention epilepsy anywhere in the script as they did not want it associated with one of their up-and-coming stars, even though it was just an acting role and integral to the plot of the film. To his credit, the late President spoke out against the ban, pointing out that it made the film hard for the audience to follow if they did not know why his character periodically had 'odd spells'.

However, things have moved on in the past 50 years and epilepsy is currently understood as a neurological condition in Western medicine, not a psychiatric disease. There is no basis for the belief that it is associated in any way with immoral conduct. The Ayurvedic explanations of the causes of epilepsy therefore appear archaic from a Western standpoint. But is there any evidence that the Ayurvedic treatment approaches are effective?

Blood-letting is invasive, painful and belongs firmly in the past as a historical treatment. There is no evidence to support blood-letting as an effective first aid technique for a seizure. The radical purging advocated by Ayurvedic practitioners will have a significant impact on the action and levels of anti-epileptic drugs in the system. In some cases, the effects of the vomiting and diarrhoea can be similar to stopping medication abruptly. More frequent, severe and prolonged seizures can result. Restarting conventional medications afterwards may not always result in the same seizure control as before.

There is evidence that some of the herbal Ayurvedic preparations used for epilepsy may have anticonvulsant properties. Examples include the processed seeds of nux-vomica, withania somnifera (ashwagandha), brahmighritham and various parts of the sesbania grandiflora plant. However, this evidence comes from laboratory studies of the chemical properties of the plants, or studies of the effects on animals specifically bred to have seizures. In the development of conventional drugs, these findings would represent the very initial stages of development of a new drug treatment. Its effectiveness would then need to be proven in a serious of well-controlled medical trials before the drug could be formally recognized and prescribed by doctors. Although Ayurvedic treatments continue to be taken by millions of people globally, there are no large scale, well-controlled trials that have looked at the effectiveness of these treatments for seizures, or have systematically monitored their safety. There have, however, been reports of worryingly high levels of arsenic in some Ayurvedic preparations. Doctors in India reported the horrifying case of an 11-year-old girl who developed signs of acute arsenic poisoning after she had been given eight Ayurvedic preparations for epilepsy. The levels of arsenic in her blood were 400 per cent greater than they should have been. Fortunately for the young girl, she recovered. However, had these effects not been discovered, further treatments would have eventually led to her death. Lead poisoning is also a real concern with some preparations.

Will it work for you?

The Ayurvedic understanding of physiology and disease is ancient. In part it presents a contrast to contemporary Western conceptions of illness and healing. Our current understanding suggests that epilepsy is a neurological rather than a psychiatric condition. It is not caused by, or associated with, immoral behaviour or attitudes. Other than the sensible Ayurvedic recommendation that 'people with epilepsy should avoid being in places where seizures could result in an injury', there is no place for invasive Ayuvedic seizure first-aid-like bloodletting in the twenty-first century. Although there is limited laboratory evidence that ingredients in some Ayurvedic medicines may have anticonvulsant properties, the purging required before these are taken is not recommended and could interfere with the effects of anti-epileptic drugs. Like other herbal preparations, Ayurvedic medicines were not regulated in the UK until May 2011. The UK government has announced that all herbal medicine practitioners will need to be regulated by the HPC in the future, but questions remain regarding the regulation of the medicines themselves. Currently, some contain dangerously high levels of poisons, including lead and arsenic. These drugs are no more 'natural' than the ones prescribed by your GP. It is difficult to see why one would choose an unproven, unregulated and possibly poisonous drug over one that has been through extensive laboratory testing, rigorous clinical trials and has been shown to be effective in controlling seizures.

9

Traditional Chinese medicine

Traditional Chinese medicine (TCM) is another ancient holistic approach to the treatment of disease. Like the majority of holistic approaches, TCM involves the concepts of a life force (qi or chi) and of balance (yin and yang). Dating back over 2500 years and a fundamental part of Chinese history and civilisation, TCM is a complex and complete system of medicine incorporating aspects of philosophy. Like the ancient Ayurvedic texts, it invokes the concept of basic elements in understanding health. In TCM there are five basic elements: wood, fire, earth, metal and water – and all are thought to be in constant flux. The five elements theory is used to interpret the relationship between the health and pathology of the human body and the natural environment. Unlike the Ayurvedic texts, which are traditionally thought to have been handed down via the gods, Chinese medicine was established through centuries of trial and error. TCM is provided in Chinese state hospitals alongside Western medicine today and its influence has spread throughout the world.

There is a strong emphasis in TCM on the prevention of illness and the maintenance of health. When illness does strike, the principle of differentiation helps a TCM practitioner to fully describe the signs of symptoms of an illness. In epilepsy, this process of differentiation extends well beyond the clinical signs considered in Western medicine and can involve a detailed examination of all aspects of an individual's lifestyle and emotional health. An analysis of these signs and symptoms within the framework of the five elements, yin and yang, and their effects on someone's vitality (qi) will result in an individualized treatment plan from the outset. This is normally based on one herb as the basic drug to treat the disease, which is then mixed with other herbs to create a multifunction formulation. This is in marked contrast to Western medicine where most people will go through a standardized procedure, initially trying one of the 'first-line' drugs at a standard dose when they are first diagnosed. In Western medicine, first-line drugs represent the first line of defence against an illness. Someone may end up with a more individualized cocktail of drugs if the first-line medications do not work and more drugs need to be added and withdrawn before they discover the right combination that works for them. But this will evolve over time, often over many years.

Chinese herbal medicine

TCM has three primary treatment methods. These are herbal medicines, acupuncture and tuina (a type of therapeutic massage). Chinese herbal medicines involve plants, minerals and animal products. The medicine prescribed will be based on the differentiation of syndrome methods unique to TCM, methods that take many years to master. Chinese herbal medicines for epilepsy may include Tianmadingxian capsules, Zhixian I pills, gouteng, shitei-to and qingyangshen. Some are simply prescribed as anti-epilepsy capsules.

What's the evidence?

Practitioners of TCM have a long tradition of clinical research and pride themselves on the scientific basis of their practice. For this reason, unlike the overwhelming majority of therapies described in this book, numerous clinical trials have been conducted to see whether TCM is an effective treatment for epilepsy. This evidence, considered alongside laboratory and animal studies, suggests that some of these herbs have anticonvulsant properties. However, almost all of these studies have, naturally, been written in Chinese and are published in Chinese medical journals. Unless you are fluent in Chinese, it is not easy to examine these reports. Fortunately, help is at hand in the shape of the Cochrane Collaboration.

The Cochrane Collaboration was established in 1993 to systematically review the evidence for the effectiveness of treatments offered around the world for all conditions. It is an international network of experts, many of whom are world leaders in their field of medicine, health policy or research methods. These experts produce completely independent reports based on rigorous criteria. When the effectiveness of any treatment for epilepsy is examined, the researchers carefully look for all of the scientific papers that have been published on the treatment. Every paper is then painstakingly examined to ensure that the study was well controlled and that no other factors could account for the findings reported by the researchers. The results of the studies that pass this rigorous scrutiny are then examined to see if there is any reliable evidence that the treatment is effective in controlling seizures and, if it is, who would be most likely to benefit. The Cochrane Collaboration works with the World Health Organization (WHO) to guide their specific health resolutions. Based on the best available evidence, healthcare providers can decide if they should fund and promote any particular treatment over and above any others. The Cochrane Library currently contains over 4500 reviews on thousands of treatments for hundreds of conditions. These reports are available in full (with a summary in plain English), free of charge to anyone who has an interest. Everyone can assess the evidence regarding the potential risks and benefits of their own treatment. Doctors also use the library to find out if a treatment is likely to be effective in a specific clinical context. (See the Useful addresses section at the end of this book for more information.) In the Cochrane Library there are over 80 reports on epilepsy treatments alone and, in 2006, the Cochrane Collaboration published their systematic review of the effectiveness of Chinese herbal medicines for epilepsy.

The Chinese researchers found 16 controlled studies of TCM for epilepsy. On the whole, the studies were not well conducted. Four studies had to be excluded from the eventual analyses as it was not clear how the participants had been diagnosed with epilepsy. Three other studies were excluded because the participants had taken Western anti-epileptic drugs in addition to the traditional Chinese herbs. In other studies, the participants were not truly randomly allocated to the treatment or the control groups. The researchers found it difficult to determine what exactly all the participants were taking in some of the studies as there were no standard doses of the active ingredient reported and the prescriptions differed widely between the patients. In the end, they found five studies that were methodologically sound enough to include in their final analysis. None involved any long-term follow-up of the participants. From the short-term data they collated, the Cochrane researchers concluded that, 'The current evidence is insufficient to support the use of traditional Chinese medicine as a treatment for epilepsy. Much larger, high quality randomized clinical trials are needed to evaluate the effectiveness and safety of traditional Chinese medicinal herbs for treating epilepsy.'

The individualized prescription of Chinese herbal medicines and general names like 'anti-epilepsy capsule' given to some of the preparations can mean that some people may not be entirely sure of what they are taking.

This is perfectly illustrated by an anecdotal case reported by Profs Schachter, Pacia and Devinsky in their book on alternative medicine for epilepsy. They recount the story of a young woman in the USA who was under the care of a neurologist but who also obtained a herbal preparation from China that she used for a short time. Shortly after she stopped taking it she ended up in her local casualty department in a very severe cluster of seizures. Blood tests found traces of phenobarbital, a powerful anti-epileptic drug that her neurologist had not prescribed. Later investigations revealed that the Chinese 'herb' contained high levels of phenobarbital. Sudden withdrawal of the drug had caused the serious deterioration in the woman's epilepsy. As the treating neurologist said, 'Quite a herb! Who knows what else it contained?'

Following an EU directive that came into force in May 2011, it is no longer possible to buy many of the more potent TCM herbal remedies directly from health food shops and other high street stockists. They will need to be prescribed by someone with a recognized qualification in TCM. Like practitioners of Ayurvedic medicine, dispensers and practioners of TCM will also need to be registered with the HPC in the future, in addition to their professional organization, if they wish to continue to prescribe many of these drugs.

Acupuncture

Acupuncture is a procedure where specific points of the body are pierced with fine needles. The places on the body that are pierced (acupuncture points) are chosen according to complex theories involving the harmonization of the five elements, yin and yang, and qi. Stimulation of these points is supposed to redress internal disharmonies and restore natural rhythms and balance. These acupuncture points lie on invisible lines and channels along the body.

In addition to traditional acupuncture with fine needles, other ways of stimulating acupuncture points have been developed, including electroacupuncture, (where pairs of acupuncture needles are attached to a machine that generates electrical pulses between them), laser acupuncture (using an extremely focused light beam instead of a needle to stimulate an acupressure point), and acupressure. In a more in-vasive procedure, 2cm lengths of sterilized cat gut are injected into acupuncture points and left there.

What's the evidence?

As with Chinese herbal medicine, there have been numerous reports in the medical literature about the possible mechanisms and effectiveness of acupuncture in epilepsy. A number of studies, in animals and humans, have found that acupuncture can cause biological responses near where the needle has been inserted and also within the brain. It is thought that the needles may stimulate the brain to release chemicals that might inhibit seizure activity.

A well-controlled study from Norway in 1999 compared acupuncture designed for epilepsy with a placebo treatment that involved the placing of needles in other points that, according to TCM theory, would not have any particular effects on seizure frequencies. All of the people in the trial had 20 treatments over the course of a month. Neither the participants in the trial nor the neurologists monitoring their seizures knew which treatment they were given. The researchers found that there was a slight reduction in the number of seizures reported in both groups but it was not statistically significant, meaning it could not reliably be attributed to the treatments. The people in the placebo group actually had more seizure-free weeks than the people who had received the genuine acupuncture. In this study, the researchers were unable to demonstrate a beneficial effect of acupuncture in people with difficult-to-treat epilepsy. A later study from the same group also failed to demonstrate any broader effects on the quality of life of people with epilepsy when using the same study design. However, other trials from China have reported more positive results.

In 2008, the Cochrane Library published their most recent review of acupuncture for epilepsy. They found 14 randomized controlled trials of acupuncture in epilepsy. Although the authors of the report say that the trials were generally of poor methodological quality (with similar criticisms as those levelled at the Chinese herbal studies), more of the acupuncture studies made it into the final analyses, with only three excluded because they did not meet the necessary standard. Disappointingly, the Cochrane authors concluded that, 'Although numerous observational human studies and experimental animal studies [suggest] potential benefits of acupuncture for treating epilepsy, there is a paucity of high quality clinical evidence. The current evidence does not support the use of acupuncture as a treatment for epilepsy.' It is, however, encouraging that no adverse effects were reported in any of these trials. Other observational studies also suggest that side effects of acupuncture are uncommon, but can occasionally include infections from needles that have not been cleaned properly. Incorrect needle placement (usually associated with novice practitioners) can occasionally cause damage to the surrounding tissue.

Tuina

Tuina is the third arm of treatment in TCM. It means 'push and grasp'. Tuina is a Chinese therapeutic massage technique that uses the meridian system and acupressure points that are used in acupuncture. The theory goes that qi can be manipulated by pushing and grasping at the points at which it gathers in the body and where the flow can become blocked. Practitioners of TCM believe that tuina is a more scientific treatment method than other kinds of massage that might simply be effective because they help to reduce stress. Since tuina massage affects not only the physical body but also the qi, TCM practitioners believe that it can have a direct impact on emotions, thoughts and spiritual well-being. Since in TCM both physical and mental health are dependant on a smooth, plentiful flow of qi, TCM practitioners believe that tuina can effectively treat many conditions.

What's the evidence?

Since tuina is an integrated part of TCM it is not often administered in isolation, but rather is part of a complete treatment package that may involve herbal medicines and acupuncture. There are no reports of any randomized controlled trials of tuina for isolation in epilepsy, and TCM regulatory bodies suggest that tuina may be most effective for tackling physical pain and musculoskeletal conditions, although original Chinese sources list over 140 medical conditions which can respond well to this form of massage. There is no clear evidence either way as to its effectiveness in epilepsy. Tuina can therefore only be judged on the rationale that underpins it.

Will it work for you?

TCM is a holistic medical approach that has an emphasis on the maintenance of health and well-being in addition to the treatment of disease. Treatments can be highly individual, with 'epilepsy' forming just part of the overall diagnosis for each individual. Although some Chinese herbal medicines have apparent anti-epileptic properties, rigorous examinations of the results of clinical trials have not found convincing evidence that they are effective. Difficulties in knowing the exact ingredients in some Chinese herbal preparations have led to some concerns regarding their safety. If you do wish to try a Chinese herbal remedy it is important that you tell whoever prescribes your anti-epileptic drugs exactly what you are, or are considering, taking. There may be harmful interactions between the Chinese herbal medicine and your regular anti-epileptic drugs which may cause the overall level of chemicals in your blood to become toxic. Never abruptly stop taking your regular medication, even if you do feel that TCMs are more effective. Only reduce your regular medications under close medical supervision.

Although there is no clear evidence that acupuncture is an effective treatment for epilepsy, it does not appear to be associated with any significant side effects. It is obviously not for you if you have a needle phobia, and many people with epilepsy already feel a bit like a pin cushion with the numerous blood tests they need to take on a regular basis. However, if the idea of qi and the unblocking of channels appeals to you, you could try tuina instead as it is based on similar principles.

This chapter ends with a couple of practical considerations. The World Wildlife Fund (WWF) has raised significant concerns about some of the animal products used in TCM. They have campaigned against the cruelty inflicted on some of the animals involved, in particular against the techniques used to collect bile from living bears. There are also significant concerns about the use of body parts from endangered animals such as black bears, tigers, rhinoceroses and seahorses in some medicines. See the WWF weblink (listed in the Useful addresses at the back of this book) for a discussion on the ethics of using these animal products in medicinal products and more on the WWF global campaign to support the use of alternatives in TCM. If you are concerned about these issues you may wish to discuss them with your TCM practitioner to ensure that these animal products are not used in any preparations you are prescribed.

In the UK, TCM has two main professional bodies: the Register of Chinese Herbal Medicine (RCHM), which has approximately 450 members, and the larger Association of Traditional Chinese Medicine (ATCM) which has more than 700 members. It is noteworthy that epilepsy is *not* listed as one of the conditions that TCM can treat on the website of either organization. If you do want to try traditional Chinese medicine always choose a practitioner who is registered with one or both of the professional bodies and with the HPC, if the regulatory legislation proposed by the UK government ever comes into force.

10

Meditation and hypnosis

Meditation

Meditation is a form of contemplation that manipulates attention. It is an ancient and fundamental part of many Eastern religions and is practised by Hindus, Buddhists and Taoists, but can also be used in a non-religious setting. There are many different types of meditation techniques. Most require complete stillness and an exclusive mental focus on one thing, such as a single featureless object, the act of breathing, the repetition of a single word or the recitation of a mantra. This eventually results in a 'loss of active attention', or a state of inattention. This state is sometimes called 'super-consciousness' and when it is associated with religious traditions it has a profound spiritual element. Meditation takes time and practice to perfect and requires regular commitment and a great deal of patience. Beginners can find the early stages of meditation unsettling and can experience fear, confusion and anxiety as disturbing thoughts and images may suddenly occur to them.

Meditation and epilepsy

The attentional changes that occur during meditation are associated with changes in the brain waves measured on an EEG. Fast, synchronized brain waves have been recorded in people in deep meditation, and these patterns remain faster, even following the meditation, than those seen in people who do not meditate. One study reported that the high-amplitude brain waves found in some experienced meditators were the highest that had ever been reported in a non-pathological context. Deep and repeated meditation clearly has the capacity to change the brain waves picked up on an EEG, but there is a fierce debate in the medical literature about whether these changes may make an epileptic seizure more or less likely to occur.

Since seizures are the results of neurons firing in a highly synchronous manner, some have argued that anything that increases these patterns within the brain may lead to an increase in the likelihood of a seizure occurring. Some have argued that seizures may even occur in people who have no previous history of epilepsy or any other known risk factors for developing the condition, if they meditate. The case of an 18-year-old young woman who practised meditation and who developed seizures was presented in a 2006 journal called *Medical Hypotheses*, as an example of just such a possibility. However, since many thousands of female 18-year-olds will develop epilepsy every year, it is likely that at least some of these young women may have an interest in meditation. In the same journal, a couple of years later, two case studies illustrating the benefits of transcendental meditation were reported. As ever, single case studies do not provide compelling evidence either way and the name of the journal that published these studies tells it all; these are just hypotheses. Theoretically, an increase in synchronous discharges within the brain may make a seizure more likely. However, the effects of stress reduction associated with meditation may make a seizure less likely. This has led to some commentators calling meditation a 'double-edged sword' in epilepsy. It is noteworthy that much of this debate between doctors and scientists has been on an entirely theoretical level: extrapolating the possible effects of the EEG changes seen in meditation to effects on the seizure thresholds of people with and without pre-existing epilepsy.

The proof of the pudding would be a well-controlled, randomized controlled trial of meditation in epilepsy. Unfortunately, it is difficult to conduct such a study, as meditation requires a great deal of personal commitment and devotion and, as such, it is not really practical to randomly allocate such a lifestyle choice to people, particularly in countries where meditation is not an integral part of the cultural landscape. Small-scale studies in India have suggested some beneficial effects on seizure control following a year of daily meditation. Exponents of the technique also point out that in actuarial tables, people who practise meditation seem to be less prone to neurological conditions than others. However, these data make no specific reference to epilepsy.

Will it work for you?

Deep meditation differs from deep relaxation and appears to result in immediate and ongoing changes in EEG patterns. Theoretically, these patterns may make seizures more likely, particularly in those who already have epilepsy. However, in practice there is no clear evidence that this is the case in countries where meditation is wide-spread. The beneficial effects of regular meditation in reducing stress are well recognized. Given that stress is a significant background trigger for a seizure in many people with epilepsy, meditation may be beneficial in this regard. As with many of the complementary and alternative therapies reviewed in this book, there are no large-scale, randomized controlled trials that have looked at the effectiveness or otherwise of meditation in controlling seizures in epilepsy; we have no solid proof either way. Meditation takes time. If it is something that appeals to you, find an experienced instructor who knows what to do if you have a seizure while you are meditating. Keep a good record of your seizures and your meditations and be aware that med-itation may result in an increase in seizures. If that appears to be the case, it may be wise to seek out another form of relaxation.

Hypnosis

Although hypnosis is often associated nowadays with the likes of Paul McKenna, Derren Brown and other stage hypnotists, it has been used as a tool for health for thousands of years. In both ancient India and Egypt, hypnotic suggestions were used as cures for a variety of conditions. It was a Scottish surgeon, James Braid, who coined the term 'hypnotism' in 1842. He rejected the magical and supernatural explanations for the feats achieved in a hypnotic state, put forward by mesmerists, and argued instead for a physio-logical explanation for the sleep-like state that hypnotism could induce. The famous French doctor, Jean Martin Charcot, working in Paris in the nineteenth century, pioneered hypnosis in the inves-tigation of hysteria. It remains a popular investigatory technique and treatment for a wide range of mental health problems to this day, and has been recognized for over 50 years by the British and American Medical Associations. Although initially wary of possible supernatural qualities, even the Vatican finally lifted its ban on hypnosis in 1956, stating that, while hypnosis is a serious matter and one not to be dabbled with, it could be used in appropriate medical settings.

Despite its relative longevity and wide acceptance, hypnosis is still not fully understood. It appears to be a state where someone can dissociate to some extent from their body and surroundings and become open to external suggestion. If the hypnotic state is deep enough they may be able to accept suggestions about their future behaviours and act on them automatically. This is called 'post-hypnotic suggestion' and forms the basis of hypnosis becoming an increasingly popular therapy for weight loss and smoking cessation.

It is perhaps unsurprising that the majority of studies of hypnotism have been on people with non-epileptic attacks rather than epilepsy. A number of studies have suggested that people with non-epileptic attacks may be more likely to have a seizure following suggestion while in a hypnotic trance, than those who have epilepsy. However, there is at least one case study in the medical literature of a person having an epileptic seizure (fully documented with EEG changes) following a regression under hypnosis to a day when he had experienced a number of seizures. So, while non-epileptic attacks may be more likely following suggestion under hypnosis, it is not totally accurate in terms of a diagnostic tool. Some of these studies also suggest that people with non-epileptic attacks may be inherently more hypnotizable than those with epilepsy.

Like meditation, hypnosis can produce significant changes in EEG activity. These changes differ depending on the task being performed under hypnosis and often represent a high state of arousal and concentration. People who are highly susceptible to hypnosis appear to differ in their EEG responses from those who are not. There is one report of a sudden death in a person with epilepsy who was brought out of a hypnotic trance very suddenly. Hypnotists experienced in working with people with epilepsy now recommend that the 'waking up' procedure should be carried out gradually so that the person does not experience a very sudden change in their level of arousal. One trial of hypnosis that paired the hypnotic state with an aromatherapy oil in 25 people with epilepsy found that, although some of the participants had a significant reduction in seizures, people who paired the aromatherapy with the relaxing state achieved via massage tended to do better than those who had been hypnotized.

Will it work for you?

Not everyone can be hypnotized. Although EEG patterns are altered during hypnosis, there is no clear evidence that it has any effect on reducing seizures in epilepsy. That is not to say it cannot be useful, just that it has not been properly evaluated in this context. Although rare, there has been one case of a sudden death following hypnosis in epilepsy. This may have been coincidental, but may be not. If you wish to pursue hypnosis for epilepsy (or any other condition) it is recommended that you seek out an experienced practitioner who is aware of the special considerations associated with hypnosis in people with epilepsy, and the need to gradually bring you out of the hypnotic state.

Autogenic training

Autogenic training is a form of self-hypnosis. It was developed in Germany in the 1920s and uses 'scripts' that people repeat to themselves to try to gain control over their body and induce a state of physical relaxation. It has been described as a kind of 'self-control therapy'. Once they have been properly taught, there is a strong emphasis on the person themselves being able to administer the therapy. The German neurologist who developed the technique believed that there was a kind of metaphorical switch within the body that people could be taught to activate themselves, inducing a hypnotic trance. Six different formulas are used to tackle different parts of the body. People are encouraged to focus on heaviness (for muscular relaxation), feelings of warmth (for vascular dilation), their heart rate, breathing, and their digestive functions. The final focus is on the forehead (for psychological calm). Imagery is encouraged as people work through fixed scripts for each area. The scripts involve calm and affirming statements such as 'I am very quiet' and 'My arms are very heavy and warm'.

There is certainly evidence that people who become proficient in autogenic training appear to be able to influence some physical processes, such as slowing their heart and breathing rates. There is some evidence that it may be effective for some conditions that are exacerbated by anxiety, such as dermatitis. But other studies have been less encouraging about its general effects in reducing stress and anxiety. As is frequently the case with alternative and complementary therapies, the studies that have been conducted have generally been poorly designed. Although autogenic training has been reported to be useful in some people with epilepsy, these reports are case studies, and no randomized controlled trials of autogenic training in people with epilepsy have been tried to date. However, intuitively it seems as though it may be an effective way to control stress. If your seizures are greatly exacerbated by stress and this approach appeals, it may be worth pursuing. Although the emphasis in autogenic training is very much on self-hypnosis, the initial training should be conducted by an experienced practitioner.

11

Aromatherapy

The way that the brain is structured reflects the way in which we evolved. Although we have been able to communicate for thousands of years, language is still quite a 'new' function in evolutionary terms. Our sense of smell is one of our oldest senses, and the parts of the brain involved in detecting aromas were among the first to develop for us as a species. This developmental pattern is also reflected in each of us individually when we are growing in the womb. The parts of the brain involved in detecting smell are those that begin to develop well before the areas that will eventually be used for language or problem solving. In the animal kingdom, scent remains critical for finding food, choosing a mate and marking out territory. A sense of smell became less important for us as a species as sight became our dominant sense. However, aromatherapy capitalizes on the fundamental way the brain responds to scent, and turns it to therapeutic advantage.

Like the herbal traditions, aromatherapy is heavily reliant on plants and their properties. However, rather than ingesting the plant whole, aromatherapy uses essential oils (highly concentrated essences) from plants, trees and flowers. These oils tend to have a strong, characteristic smell depending on the plant from which they have been extracted. The healing and preserving properties of these oils have been recognized at various points through history. The ancient Egyptians used these oils to embalm and preserve their dead. It did not take long for the women of the time to use the same oils to try to preserve their skin while they were alive, a preoccupation that continues to this day. During London's Great Plague of 1665, apothecaries and their assistants appeared to have relative immunity from the Black Death, attributed in part to the antiseptic qualities of the essential oils they were working with on a daily basis. In the late nineteenth century, a French chemist named

Gattefosse burnt his hand in an explosion in his laboratory. In agony, he instinctively plunged his hand into the nearest liquid, which happened to be a vat of lavender oil. To his amazement, his pain was greatly reduced and his hand healed, apparently without scarring. In the Second World War another Frenchman, surgeon Jean Valnet, used Gattefosse's experiences to champion the use of essential oils to aid the postoperative healing in soldiers wounded in battle. He later used the oils and their aromas to treat psychiatric disorders.

Today, aromatherapy is used to treat a variety of disorders from high blood pressure to insomnia, headaches to skin conditions. The oils can be used in a bath, massaged into the skin, inhaled through a diffuser or taken as a tincture. Aromatherapists attribute certain characteristics to different oils – some are seen as reviving (for example, cypress, sage, lemongrass, rosemary, bergamot), while others are viewed as calming (chamomile, lavender, sandalwood, ylang ylang, jasmine). Some essential oils are purported to improve memory functions (lemon, anise, rosemary, peppermint, sage). It is no coincidence that many of the conditions most frequently targeted by aromatherapists have a strong association with anxiety and are greatly exacerbated by stress. Aromatherapy can also be used to treat epilepsy.

How does it work?

There are three ways in which aromatherapy may be effective in reducing seizures in some people with epilepsy.

The first is via the anticonvulsant properties of the oils themselves. Some oils appear to have anticonvulsant properties when they enter the bloodstream. In animal studies, seizure thresholds were raised in rats who were fed essential oil of lemongrass. Any seizures they did have were also less prolonged than when they had not been fed the oil. Other essential oils with possible anticonvulsant properties include jasmine and ylang ylang. Very small quantities of these oils may also enter the bloodstream if they are absorbed through the skin via massage, or inhaled. Some have argued that since these methods bypass any processing by the gastrointestinal system, the effects on the brain chemistry may be more potent. While this may be the case in theory, the effect is probably mitigated by the very small amounts involved. Nevertheless, it would be wise for people with epilepsy to avoid inhaling some of the essential oils that may have proconvulsant qualities (that is they may make a seizure more likely to occur), particularly those that have high levels of camphor – these include rosemary, fennel, sage, hyssop and wormwood.

If the direct chemical effects of the essential oils on brain chemistry are small when absorbed through the skin or inhaled, then how else might aromatherapy be beneficial for seizures? The second way is via conditioning. Conditioning is a psychological phenomena that was first described in 1901 by a Russian physiologist named Pavlov. In his experiments with dogs he noticed that they began to salivate at the sight of their food being prepared, and at him bringing the food to them. He then rang a bell every time their food was being prepared. The dogs soon learnt to associate the sound of the bell with food and would salivate whenever they heard the bell, regardless of whether food came along or not. The technique of associating an arbitrary event with an automatic behaviour is called conditioning. It is a very powerful and remarkably robust technique. All kinds of natural human responses can be 'conditioned' to artificial stimuli. Many aspects of your own behaviours will have been conditioned without you being consciously aware of it. Advertisers use these principles all the time to pair their chosen images and sounds with feelings.

Likewise, aromatherapy can be used to associate particular states of mind with specific smells. If aromatherapy is used via massage or with active relaxation techniques over a number of sessions, the brain will begin to associate that smell with a sense of calm and tranquillity. The smell can then be used when someone begins to feel anxious and stressed, to try to help them regain the feelings of calm. In epilepsy this technique can be used as soon as someone gets a warning or a sense that a seizure is about to happen, in an attempt to 'divert' the brain away from a seizure and towards the state that is associated with the smell.

Even without the previous pairing of specific aromas with psychological states, there is some evidence that just the experience of some very strong smells can interfere with seizure activity in the brain. This is the third way in which aromatherapy may be helpful in epilepsy. Seizures occur when the neurons begin to fire abnormally together and become synchronized. The experience of a strong odour can break this pattern, forcing the neurons to desynchronize. A number of newer treatments for epilepsy, such as vagal nerve stimulation (VNS), and thalamic stimulation (a new kind of brain surgery), are also thought to work, in part due to the effects they have on de-synchronizing the neurons, making them less likely to fire abnormally together. As such, strong smells have recently been advocated as both a pre-emptive treatment to prevent seizures and as a possible intervention to arrest seizure activity for some people, particularly those with temporal lobe epilepsy.

Traditional folk remedies for epilepsy that are widespread in the Indian subcontinent are very interesting in this regard. Many people from this region grow up believing that seizures can be aborted by wafting an old shoe under the sufferer's nose. The smellier the shoe, the better. While the roots of this remedy appear to lie in the belief that the vile smell would draw out the evil spirits that were causing the seizure (a case of like attracting like), it is possible that the longevity of the tradition and its continued popularity today may be based on the very real physical associations between a sense of smell and temporal lobe epilepsy.

What's the evidence?

As with many of the complementary and alternative therapies reviewed in this book, there are numerous case studies of individuals who have experienced a significant reduction in seizure control following a course of aromatherapy.

The Birmingham trial

However, unlike many of the other therapies, there is also some evidence that it may be an effective treatment. A trial of aromatherapy in 100 people with epilepsy was conducted at an NHS hospital in Birmingham by a team of epilepsy doctors. The setting is important because they ensured that all of the people enrolled on the trial had a clear diagnosis of epilepsy. Often, a criticism of studies that do not involve medical doctors is that the people involved may not actually have epilepsy and may be suffering from non-epileptic attacks. That is not the case in this study. The researchers used aromatherapy massage on six occasions over the course of three weeks and encouraged the participants to associate the smell of the oil with the relaxed feeling they got from the massage. The participants then practised just smelling the oil (without the massage) in order to relax and were also encouraged to smell the oil if they felt that a seizure was about to happen, or if they were in a situation where they felt a seizure was more likely to occur. They also placed a drop of the oil on their pillow three times a week prior to going to sleep. The results of the trial were remarkable with one in three people completely seizure-free one year after the treatment began. Another third experienced a reduction of at least 50 per cent in their seizure frequencies. The researchers were cautious about these results and point out that many factors may have also played a part in the improvements recorded, including the development of a basic proficiency in relaxation and stress management techniques; nevertheless, the results are very encouraging. In this study, the participants were allowed to choose their own oils, based on the aromas they liked. Interestingly, all opted for one of the oils that is reputed to lower arousal (jasmine, ylang ylang, lavender, camomile, bergamot or marjoram). The researchers felt that jasmine may have been the most effective oil, but were at pains to point out that this was a tentative finding.

Some people do not like the very distinctive smell of jasmine. If that is the case for you, another oil from the soothing category that you do find pleasant is likely to be more effective.

Will it work for you?

There is a sound scientific basis to support the use of aromatherapy in epilepsy. In fact, the theory behind it suggests that it may work in a number of ways. Although the gold standard of a randomized control trial of aromatherapy in epilepsy is yet to be conducted, there is some reasonably convincing evidence that it may work for some people, particularly those with temporal lobe epilepsy. People with epilepsy should avoid contact with some oils that have high concentrations of camphor as they may actually make a seizure more likely. However, aromatherapy that pairs a distinctive smell, such as jasmine, with a relaxed state may be helpful in reducing seizures. Although scarce, the evidence that is available suggests that the benefits of aromatherapy massage may be long-lasting and, in time, exposure to just the scent itself may be sufficient to reduce the number of seizures.

Aromatherapy is offered by some NHS trusts for some conditions, such as maternity care, but is not widely available for epilepsy. The costs for six sessions will vary, dependent upon where you live. Aromatherapy massage involves some body exposure and some people may not feel comfortable with this. If that is the case, then you are unlikely to find an aromatherapy massage a relaxing experience. You may be able to find another way to pair the smell of your chosen oil with a relaxed state, for example as an infusion in the bath. However, this will probably be less effective than massage as the oils are also absorbed into the body via the skin as well via the olfactory system during massage. The aromatherapy programme that produced the best results in the NHS Birmingham trial demanded time and dedication from the participants; they were not just the passive recipients of a few massages. Nevertheless, the results were encouraging, and if you are prepared to put the effort in, the evidence available does suggest that this may be a promising approach to try. A final word of caution: unfortunately, aromatherapy may not work for you if you have a poor sense of smell.

12

Physical manipulation therapies: chiropractic care and craniosacral therapy

Chiropractic care

Like many of the therapies that are grouped under the complementary and alternative medicine umbrella, chiropractic care is another treatment based on a holistic view of health and wellness. Diseases and symptoms are not viewed as distinct and separate entities but in the context of the whole person. Chiropractic was developed by Daniel David Palmer, a Canadian 'magnetic healer' in the late nineteenth century. He was an active spiritualist and developed the ideas that eventually became chiropractic, via spiritual messages apparently received from a dead doctor. He reasoned that the spine must be involved in most illnesses, because that was the structure that connected the head to the body. He thought that misalignments in this core connection would cause problems in distant parts of the body and therefore concluded that by correcting these misalignments, the remote symptoms would resolve. He stated that, 'A subluxated vertebra . . . is the cause of 95 per cent of all diseases . . . The other five per cent is caused by displaced joints other than those of the vertebral column.' Some of his very first cases included treatment of a man who was deaf and another who had a heart condition.

The primary mode of treatment offered by modern chiropractors today is spinal manipulation and over 100 different techniques are employed. These manipulations are primarily used to treat neck and back pain with the notion of correcting various conditions of aberrant motion or function. However, by the early twenty-first century there had been a gradual, and rather controversial, creep of the technique into the treatment of other non-musculoskeletal conditions. In 2001, one study found that non-musculoskeletal complaints accounted for over 10 per cent of the chief complaints presented to chiropractors in the USA.

This is a controversial therapy and there are many different views about how effective it is. These conflicting views have in the past sparked a fierce media debate and given rise to the 'Sense About Science' campaign. (See the Useful addresses at the back of this book for more information.)

What's the evidence?

There is no scientific basis for a role of chiropractic care in the treatment of epilepsy. Although a few case studies have been written up of people's seizures responding to spinal manipulation, there is little to distinguish these responses from natural variations in the course of someone's epilepsy. While poorly documented, anecdotal, reports of a gradual improvement in seizure control following spinal adjustments cannot be considered proof of an effective treatment, well documented case studies of serious side effects following such manipulations must be taken seriously.

Manipulation of the neck can cause damage to the arteries which supply the brain. If this damage is severe it can lead to stroke, and in rare cases, death.

Laurie Mathiason

In 1998, Laurie Mathiason was a 20-year-old Canadian waitress who visited a chiropractor complaining of stiffness in her neck. That evening she became increasingly uncoordinated and returned to the chiropractor for further manipulations. She suffered a seizure during the treatment and was rushed to hospital where she slipped into a coma. She died three days later. The coroner's report documented that Laurie had 'died of a ruptured vertebral artery, which occurred in association with a chiropractic manipulation of the neck'. Although rare, this case is not unique.

In summary, there is no scientific rationale behind the use of chiropractic manipulations in the treatment of epilepsy. The mechanisms that have been suggested are simply untested ideas. Similarly, there is no solid clinical evidence that it is an effective treatment for seizure disorders. However, there is some all too real and tragic evidence that it may, in rare cases, disrupt the flow of blood to the brain. This can result in seizures, stroke, coma and death. It is difficult to imagine that one would want to run these risks, however small, in the absence of any clear rationale as to why it would work, or evidence that it is helpful for someone with epilepsy.

Craniosacral therapy

Craniosacral therapy was developed by Dr William Sutherland in the early twentieth century. He believed that the bones of the skull were moveable and that specific emotions and pain could be elicited from a person if pressure was placed upon the right places on the skull. He also believed that he could teach people to self-correct the movements of skull bones in a therapeutic fashion to address specific ailments. Nowadays, there remains a great deal of scepticism among anatomists as to whether cranial bones do move, and if they do, whether such small movements can have any therapeutic effects.

Nevertheless, by applying very light fingertip pressure to the skull, craniosacral therapists claim that they can detect alternating 'rhythms' in individual brain lobes. These craniosacral rhythms can be 'palpated' by changing the fingertip pressures on the skull. The therapists claim that these rhythms feel 'sluggish' or 'ratcheting' in people with epilepsy. Some even claim to be able to identify scar tissue within the brain.

Such claims of sensitivity to brain structure and function via fingertips on a skull fall well outside the known laws of natural science and border on the supernatural. They are also unproven. Unsurprisingly, studies that have looked at the reliability of different craniosacral therapists in detecting the craniosacral rhythms have found no consistency between them. There is no scientific evidence that such an approach is effective in treating epilepsy.

Will it work for you?

Therapies that involve the manipulation of the spine or skull have been promoted by some practitioners as beneficial for epilepsy. Such applications of chiropractic care are not recommended for epilepsy by the British Chiropractic Association and there is no scientific evidence that they work. Likewise, there is no scientific basis for the use of craniosacral therapy for seizure disorders.

13

Homoeopathy

Homoeopathy was developed in the early 1800s by a German doctor called Samuel Hahnemann. By experimenting on himself with some of the cures for malaria at the time, he noticed that one of the apparent cures actually seemed to cause some of the symptoms of the disease. Shortly after taking a preparation of a tree bark, he began to experience a fever with shivering, aches and pains. We now know that the bark he ingested contained the anti-malarial compound, quinine, and taking quinine in moderate doses can cause a condition called 'cinchonism' (also known as 'quininism') in some people. Symptoms of cinchonism include sweating, headaches and stomach upsets. Hahnemann concluded that all the effective drugs used to treat sick people would induce a mild form of the illness they were supposed to treat if they were taken by healthy people. These ideas were eventually developed into the 'law of similars' or 'let like be cured by like' – a concept that continues to underpin the theoretical foundations of homoeopathy to this day.

By 1810, Hahnemann had identified 65 remedies for many conditions and symptoms, including epilepsy. All were developed by observing the physical symptoms caused by various substances taken by himself and other people who were healthy. Subsequent practitioners have continued his work and today there are over 4000 homoeopathic remedies on offer, with 240 specifically designed for seizures. Rather than treating specific disease entities like epilepsy, homoeopaths take a more holistic view of the symptoms people experience. Each symptom or complaint is seen within the context of a disturbance in the 'life force' of the individual, and some take a very spiritual view of this 'life force'. A homoeopathic consultation, therefore, is normally very thorough, involving a detailed discussion and examination of many aspects of an individual's personal, social and emotional life, in addition to their physical complaints. The remedy or remedies that are eventually prescribed will be chosen specifically for the individual as a whole, based on the homoeopath's understanding of the patient's mind, body and spirit, not just as a response to the presenting 'disease'. As a result, different people with the same condition, such as epilepsy, may be prescribed different remedies.

How is it supposed to work?

Hahnemann believed that if large doses of a substance produced specific symptoms, the same substance would, in extremely small doses, cure them. In an effort to create the smallest possible doses, he began to dilute substances to create homoeopathic 'remedies'. Hahnemann advocated dilution of the original substance to the extent that the resultant remedy would only contain one part of the original substance to one trillion (1,000,000,000,000) parts of the solution in which it has been diluted. In fact, in direct contrast to modern medicines, homoeopaths continue to believe that the more dilute a substance is, the more potent it will be.

The idea that 'like can treat like' is just that, an idea. It has no scientific basis. The homoeopathic 'law of similars' should not be confused with the principle that underlies vaccination in conventional medicine. In vaccination, the body is injected with either an inactivated or significantly weakened organism with no, or very little, potential for real harm, in order to 'teach' the body to recognize the organism as a threat, so it can respond rapidly if it encounters the real thing in the future. This is very different from using a substance that creates symptoms as a treatment. The idea that 'less is more' may work when promoting minimalist fashion and food trends, but it contravenes many of the natural laws of physics when it comes to the effects of physical substances. Hahnemann drew up his recommended dilution strengths believing that dilution could be infinite. This was before scientists found out that molecules existed and that they were of a certain size. We now know that dilution cannot be infinite, as after a while there will be no molecules of the original substance left in the solution. The huge numbers involved in homoeopathic dilutions are mind boggling and modern critics of homoeopathy have a great deal of fun creating analogies for the 'strength' of the remedies prescribed. Dr Ben Goldacre, a GP, journalist and outspoken critic of homoeopathy, suggests in his entertaining book, *Bad Science*, that one should imagine a giant bubble of water with a diameter of 150 million kilometres (that is roughly the distance between the earth and the sun). One molecule of the active substance within that sphere of water would represent what is known as a 30C homoeopathic remedy, and that is a relatively dense solution in homoeopathic terms, where dilutions of 200C are readily available. Dr Goldacre's scathing criticisms are not new. As early as 1843, Queen Victoria's personal doctor described the theory behind homoeopathy as 'an outrage to human reason', and yet many people even today, including high profile celebrities and some in the highest echelons of the royal family, swear by it as a valuable, effective treatment for a whole range of conditions. Could it somehow work despite its nonsensical scientific underpinnings?

What's the evidence?

In 2010, the UK government completed an enquiry into whether homoeopathic medicine should be available on the NHS. The House of Commons Science and Technology Committee concluded that there was no convincing evidence that homoeopathy worked, other than having a placebo effect, and that it should not be funded by the NHS for any condition. A fierce public debate ensued. Currently, some NHS funding for homoeopathic treatment continues, under the guise of ensuring that patients have choice in their treatment. However, the debate rages on as to whether this is even a valid choice for people to make, in the face of a distinct lack of any scientific evidence that it works or a credible rationale as to why it should.

There have been no randomized, controlled trials of homoeopathic remedies in epilepsy to date. There is, therefore, no scientific evidence that it is an effective treatment for the condition. Proponents of homoeopathy argue that the lack of trials is due to difficulties in finding funding to conduct these studies together with a myriad of other methodological difficulties. They also point to numerous case studies where homoeopathy appears to have a beneficial effect on seizure control. Unfortunately for the homeopaths, case studies count for little more than anecdotal evidence in the quest for scientific proof. As Chapter 2 explained, many people have good and bad spells with their epilepsy and the onset of good spells will inevitably coincide with new treatment regimes for some. The emphasis here is on coincide; it is often a coincidence.

Will it work for you?

The UK government committee concluded that homoeopathy was a placebo. They went further and suggested that prescribing a pure placebo was bad medicine and that it could not form the sole basis of any treatment on the NHS. This is certainly true if it were the only treatment offered, but what about in combination with other treatments? We know that the so-called placebo effect is a real phenomenon that produces tangible, replicable results (see Chapter 2). People receiving placebos do better than those who receive no treatment at all. In terms of the attributes that a placebo needs to maximize its effectiveness, homoeopathy ticks all of the boxes. The remedy is prescribed by a practitioner who has a firm belief that it works. The homoeopath conducts a very thorough, deeply personal interview with the patient, asking them about almost every aspect of their lives, including events, sensations, memories, dreams, emotions and thoughts. Their deep interest in the person with epilepsy is an integral part of creating the remedy. The rituals surrounding the preparation of the remedy are elaborate, shrouded in metaphysical concepts, and the result is a bespoke treatment in a bottle. If someone were to pull together all of the scientific data on the placebo effect and create the optimal approach, it would look very like homoeopathy.

Nowhere is this more clearly illustrated than in a leafy quiet square in the heart of London. This is home to a hospital housed in a smart, clean, cream building with a light and spacious modern interior. Someone with epilepsy attending this hospital will be the absolute centre of care and attention while the homoeopathic practitioner takes a more detailed history than they will have ever experienced in a traditional neurology clinic or in the six minutes normally allotted to them at their NHS GP surgery. After a long face-to-face consultation, they will leave with a medicine specifically chosen and designed not just for their symptoms but one that takes into account their wider circumstances too.

In the same square is a hospital which is the base for a world-class group of epilepsy doctors and scientists. This is an old, Victorian red brick building, and on entering, someone with epilepsy is immediately confronted by dark wood and NHS green walls as they head for the crowded, windowless, outpatient waiting room. They may wait (sometimes for hours) to see their consultant who will be under immense pressure to get them out of the door as soon as possible in order to see the next patient and to stop the clinic overrunning even longer. The doctor may prescribe a new medication but will be at pains to point out that the chances of it working at this point in their condition may be 10 per cent or less. Not all NHS consultations are like this of course. This is a worse case scenario, but you can guess which person with epilepsy would probably feel better about their condition and more in control as they both leave their respective hospitals and make their way home across the square.

So, while a homoeopathic remedy will not work on the basis of the ideological basis upon which it was developed, many features of the treatment may confer benefits upon people suffering from a variety of conditions, including epilepsy. If you believe in the metaphysical explanations, all the better.

While adding homoeopathic remedies to your anti-epileptic treatment regime may have some beneficial effects, if nothing more than a temporary effect on your general sense of well-being and being cared for, it is important to remember that homoeopathic remedies should *never* be used as the sole treatment for epilepsy. Even if your seizures appear to be fully controlled by a new remedy you should not stop taking your anti-epileptic medications without consulting your doctor. To do so be can be very dangerous. Most reputable homoeopathic practitioners recognize this and it is worth seeking out a medically qualified homoeopath if you wish to pursue the possibility of a homoeopathic remedy for your seizures. Medically qualified homoeopaths recognize the importance of conventional medicines in treating serious conditions and use homoeopathy as an add-on therapy. They are also more likely than lay practitioners to spot any serious underlying conditions that may need additional medical intervention.

It is fitting to conclude this chapter with the words of one such medically qualified homoeopath, Dr John Hughes-Games, a GP, who was the former president of the faculty of homoeopathy at the Bristol Homeopathic Hospital. He was appalled by the disastrous, sometimes fatal, consequences of lay homoeopathy in cases where serious illnesses had failed to be diagnosed by non-medical professionals. The importance of a bedrock of full medical training became part and parcel of his energetic promotion of the homoeopathic approach as an add-on therapy. He commanded such respect and loyalty that when he lay dying of cancer in his NHS hospital bed in 2004 and was unable to see the birds and the sky through the dirty hospital windows, he raised enough money from his patients and colleagues to have all of the hospital windows cleaned for the benefit of every patient. Before Dr Hughes-Games died he wrote the following:

The best way to recover from an illness would be to have someone or something evoke [a] healing response – no drugs, no knives – splendid! Indeed if homeopathy were only a superb way of producing a placebo response, its existence would be more than justified by that alone.

14

Light therapy

In ancient civilizations across the globe, the sun and the moon were often believed to hold significant powers over humans. The sun god in each tradition was normally associated with power, omnipotence and strength, and much had to be done to appease and please him to ensure that he re-appeared each day. Mass sun-worship nowadays is mostly restricted to those who like to bake themselves on crowded beaches for aesthetic purposes. But many continue to believe that the moon and planets can have a significant influence on their health, wealth and happiness, hence the continued popularity of horoscopes and astrology. While there is no evidence to support astrological interpretations of seizure occurrence based on star signs or arbitrary planetary conjunctions, some reputable studies have found a relationship between phases of the lunar cycle and patterns of seizures in large groups of people with epilepsy.

However, there is little consistency between the reports and they probably reflect the fact that if 20 people look for a significant pattern, one of them might just find a chance grouping that looks significant, but is not. Some blue-sky thinkers have suggested that the gravitational effect of the moon could exert an influence on the water mass in our bodies (in the same way that it affects the tides). Others have suggested that the moon could somehow affect cerebral function via changes in the earth's electromagnetic field. Even if these effects were proven, it takes a leap of pure speculation to think that this might affect seizure thresholds. However, there is a way that the moon might affect the likelihood that someone may have a seizure. One study found that the brightness of the moon did appear to be related to the number of seizures that occurred in an inpatient ward for people with epilepsy. If the moon was full and it was a cloudless night, then more people had seizures in the following 24 hours than on moonless nights, or nights when the moonlight was obscured by heavy cloud cover. Since an earlier study had found that people, on average, slept 20 minutes less during the full moon phase, and that their morning fatigue was greater, the epilepsy researchers concluded that sleep deprivation and disruption to the normal sleep–wake cycle associated with a bright night was probably the most likely explanation for an increase in seizure activity associated with the lunar cycle.

The development of light therapy

The possibilities of using light as a therapy for epilepsy initially came from doctors' casual observations that people being treated in a dedicated epilepsy unit tended to have fewer seizures on sunny days than on dull, overcast days. So they logged all the seizures that happened over the course of a year on the ward and looked to see if there really was a relationship between the number of sunshine hours and the number of seizures recorded. Sure enough, they found a significant correlation.

If sunlight does affect seizure thresholds and make it less likely that someone will have a seizure, the doctors reasoned that this pattern would be reflected in the rates of epilepsy reported in different countries. Unfortunately, there is no data on the average number of seizures people with epilepsy experience in each country, but there is some information on the proportion of the population in each country who have a diagnosis of epilepsy. There are many difficulties in comparing these rates of epilepsy in different countries since some studies may include children and older people and others may exclude them. Also the very different standards of healthcare available to people around the world mean that the data that is available may underestimate rates in some developing countries. There are also some regional influences that make some places 'hot spots' for some types of epilepsy. Epilepsy can result from encephalitis, a term that covers a wide variety of diseases that cause the brain to become irritated and swollen. Encephalitis is generally more common in tropical regions, and epilepsy hotspots have developed in communities with high levels of HIV infection, or inadequate vaccination programmes. The Lassa virus is widespread in rodents that live throughout sub-Saharan and West Africa. It is transmitted to people via contact with faeces or urine from infected rodents or via dust containing infective particles and is responsible for many cases of epilepsy in the region. The pork tapeworm likes to use the human brain as a nursery for its larvae. This causes seizures. In parts of the world where food hygiene is not good, these larvae may be responsible for local 'outbreaks' of epilepsy.

With all these complex regional factors that influence the prevalence of epilepsy in any given population, it is very difficult to isolate any effects of the weather or climate in different countries. But, remarkably, there is some evidence to suggest that baseline levels of epilepsy may be lower in countries nearer the equator than further north, when regional factors are accounted for. Within Europe, too, there is some evidence that epilepsy is less common in the sunnier southern European countries like Spain and Italy compared to Scandinavia.

The importance of vitamin D

Having established that people in the UK tend to have fewer seizures on sunny days and that people in sunnier countries may have lower rates of epilepsy, the doctors began to look at why sunlight might affect seizure thresholds in people with epilepsy. Light is important for us in two main respects. Sunlight is a very important source of vitamin D; in fact, we get over 90 per cent of our vitamin D from exposure to sunlight and only about 10% from our food. Vitamin D is important for bone health and growth and severe deficiencies can lead to rickets, a condition that is once again on the rise in the UK. It can also lead to seizures. It is estimated that more than half of the UK population do not get enough vitamin D. Vitamin D deficiencies are even more common in people with epilepsy who take anti-epileptic drugs, as some of these medications appear to inhibit the natural production of vitamin D.

So, sunlight can boost vitamin D levels, which in turn can raise seizure thresholds. Sunlight also plays a part in regulating melatonin levels. Melatonin is a hormone that regulates our sleeping and waking cycle every day. Levels of melatonin rise in the evening, when the natural light goes, to prepare us for sleep. We begin to feel sleepy and some body systems slow down in the presence of melatonin. Exposure to natural light in the morning turns off the production of melatonin and the systems wake up again. If this daily cycle of melatonin production gets disrupted, people can develop sleep problems. Melatonin also plays an important role in regulating seizure thresholds but the relationship is complex. It is not simply a question of adding melatonin, like a drug, although this has been tried in some children. What does seem clear is that it is the cycle of the melatonin that needs to be preserved, to ensure that seizure thresholds are breached as infrequently as possible.

The evidence suggests that sunlight might be an important factor in regulating seizure thresholds. This is backed up by clinical observations of the patterns of seizures that occur on an epilepsy ward, patterns of the prevalence of epilepsy around the world, and also scientific studies of the effects of light on the brain. But could this knowledge be converted into a useful treatment for epilepsy?

Sunshine is a significant source of vitamin D because ultra violet (UV) rays from sunlight trigger vitamin D synthesis in the skin. Most artificial sources of light try to avoid UV rays as they can damage the skin in concentrated forms. The best way to boost vitamin D levels for people is therefore through increasing natural exposure of the skin to the sun and maximizing intake through diet and vitamin D supplements (see Chapter 6).

While artificial sources of light may not produce vitamin D, they can be very useful in helping to regulate the daily cycle of melatonin. Light boxes have been used for many years to do just that in people with seasonal affective disorder (SAD), sometimes called 'winter blues'. This is a depressive illness that affects people in the winter months. Daily exposure to a strong, bright light in the morning can help lift the mood in people with SAD and is widely recognized as one of the most effective treatments for this condition. Scientists are beginning to realise that there are strong links between epilepsy and depression and the common systems they affect in the brain. One fascinating finding is that depression appears to predate the onset of epilepsy in many people. Previously, doctors have just thought that people were depressed because they had been given a diagnosis of epilepsy, but this finding suggests that the two conditions may share common biological links. Studies of the effects of light on brain chemistry indicate that it can influence the chemical systems involved in the regulation of mood and seizures. In 2011, the first randomized controlled trial of light therapy in epilepsy was conducted.

What's the evidence?

One hundred people took part in the study. Half were given a high-intensity light box, identical to those used to treat seasonal affective disorder, and half were allocated a low-intensity light box. The participants were asked to sit in front of the box for 20 minutes each morning for three months. Its not as arduous as it sounds, as they were able to do other things at the same time, like eating breakfast, checking their emails, and watching the television. The researchers compared the number of seizures they experienced on the days when they had used the box to those when they had not. The results of the trial were mixed. While some people with temporal lobe seizures had a significant reduction in their seizures, others, particularly those with seizures that came from other regions of the brain, derived no significant benefits, and for some it made their seizures worse. For the people who did experience a benefit, there was a significant relationship between the number of times they used the box and the number of seizures they experienced, with fewer seizures occurring in those who used the box most regularly. Although the effects of the light-box treatment were mixed when it came to seizure control, the treatment had a significant positive impact on the participants' mood and levels of anxiety. Some participants also recorded that the light box helped them combat some of the morning fatigue associated with their anti-epileptic medications.

Will it work for you?

Light box therapy is a new treatment for epilepsy. Although the theory has a sound scientific basis, so far there has only been one trial of light therapy in epilepsy and the results were mixed. Regular use of a light box may reduce the frequency of focal and secondary generalized seizures for some people with temporal lobe epilepsy, but more studies are needed to confirm these findings. Light therapy may also help to improve low mood and reduce anxiety in people with epilepsy. Many people may prefer to try this non-invasive treatment for low mood before adding antidepressants to the many anti-epileptic medications they may already be taking. There is anecdotal evidence that suggests that the use of a light box may help combat some of the morning fatigue and difficulties in getting going in the morning that some people with epilepsy experience associated with their medications.

People with generalized epilepsy should use a light box with caution. It may make their seizures worse. At present, there is only evidence to suggest that it may help people with temporal lobe epilepsy.

Light boxes are not available from the NHS and are not normally covered by private health insurance. There are many companies selling them on the internet and as a result they are gradually coming down in price. However, very cheap models may not emit enough light for them to work on a therapeutic basis. Generally, the lower the intensity of the light, the longer someone has to sit in front of it in the morning to get a therapeutic dose. High-powered light boxes (emitting 10,000 lux) generally require 20 to 30 minutes exposure and may cost around £200. Some companies offer the option of renting a light box on a monthly basis, which may be useful if you want to see if it does work for you, before you make a larger financial commitment. It is worth reiterating that the evidence to date suggests that a light box may require more than a financial commitment to maximize the chances of success. The data from the trial suggested that it was the people who were able to use it every day who derived the most benefit. You may need to think carefully about your daily routine to ensure that you have enough time in the morning to accommodate this therapy. Wall brackets, desk mounts and portable versions are available to help incorporate the light therapy into your everyday routine. Light boxes should not be confused with dawn simulators (alarm clocks with a light that comes on gradually in the morning). Blue light boxes that emit blue light have been designed to be easier on the eyes, but as yet there is no evidence either way of their effectiveness for mood or seizure control in people with epilepsy.

15

Oxygen

All of the cells in our body need oxygen to function properly and our brain cells are voracious consumers. Oxygen is transported to the cells via the blood stream. The average concentration of oxygen in the blood is normally about 95 per cent, but this can change when people are unwell or when the amount of oxygen in the air they are breathing is greater or lower than normal. The amount of oxygen in the air we breathe is dependent on air pressure. The lack of oxygen at high altitude is one of the greatest challenges for mountaineers. At the top of Mount Everest there is approximately 65 per cent less oxygen in the air than at sea level. Air under greater pressure than that experienced at sea level, for example under the sea, is more dense. Hyperbaric oxygen (HBO) chambers are devices that use these physical properties of air pressure to deliver higher densities of oxygen to people for therapeutic purposes. The procedure takes place in a sealed chamber and the oxygen can be delivered via a hood for around an hour at a time. Participants normally notice a change in pressure in their ears, similar to that experienced in an aircraft. Different treatment regimes are recommended for different conditions, but most involve upwards of 30 regular (daily) sessions of around 60 minutes.

Deep sea divers are familiar with HBO chambers as they are used very effectively to treat 'the bends', a condition that develops if a diver surfaces too rapidly. However, HBO therapy has also been recommended to speed up healing in a number of other conditions, including infections, skin grafts, burns and crush injuries. There is much written on the internet about the possibilities of HBO for epilepsy, but the scientific evidence reveals that HBO can actually cause seizures, rather than prevent them.

What's the evidence?

HBO therapy provides extra oxygen in the blood. Neurons can become starved of oxygen (hypoxic) in some conditions, and this can sometimes occur during or after a prolonged seizure. While HBO therapy will provide hypoxic neurons with much-needed oxygen, it may actually induce seizures if the neurons are in a normal state, even in someone without any previous history of epilepsy. Scientists have known for over 200 years that breathing in pure oxygen causes seizures. Increased oxygen intake via HBO can cause an initial constriction followed by a sudden surge in the blood flow in the brain, which can trigger a seizure. Nitric oxide is produced by neurons during HBO therapy and this also increases brain blood flow, which can precipitate a seizure. There is evidence from animal studies that repeated exposure to HBO therapy increases the epileptic sensitivity of rats, and after a while they begin to have seizures earlier and earlier in the HBO treatment sessions.

Regardless of these concerns, some have used HBO as a direct treatment for epilepsy. A Chinese study from the Eleventh International Congress on Hyperbaric Medicine in 1987 is widely cited and referenced on the internet in this regard. Unfortunately, this study, reporting remarkable improvements in seizure control recorded in over 80 per cent of the children with epilepsy who took part, has not been presented for peer review in an international medical journal and so it is impossible to examine the basis of the claims. It is, however, a neat case study that highlights the 'viral' nature of the way information spreads across the internet.

HBO is an emerging experimental treatment for children with cerebral palsy, many of whom may have epilepsy as well. In two well designed, peer-reviewed, randomized control trials of HBO, researchers have failed to find a significant effect on behavioural and cognitive measures in children with cerebral palsy who received the HBO therapy compared to those in the placebo group. The only significant differences between the two groups in one study was an increase in ear problems in the group that had received the HBO therapy. There are also a number of case reports in the medical literature of serious complications following HBO in children with cerebral palsy, including generalized tonic clonic seizures induced in a ten-month-old boy, caused by an undissolved oxygen bubble that went to his brain and caused a stroke.

Will it work for you?

There is no scientific evidence to support the use of HBO therapy in epilepsy. Basic science and experimental work in animals suggests that HBO therapy may actually increase the risk of seizures. A number of case studies have linked the onset of seizures to HBO therapy in people without a previous history of epilepsy. The evidence to date suggests that HBO is not an effective treatment for people with epilepsy and that it may actually aggravate the propensity to experience seizures.

16

Neurofeedback

Biofeedback is a technique that displays information about otherwise 'hidden' biological functions, in an effort to help someone gain control over them. For example, scientists have shown that people can learn to have some control over their heart rate. Natural increases and decreases in heart rate can be monitored and displayed back on TV monitors. Over time, people may begin to recognize some of the previously subconscious factors that are associated with these fluctuations. Feelings of anxiety or excitement may accompany an increase in heart rate while feelings of relaxation may be associated with reduced heart rate. If small rewards are offered for desired heart rates and punishments are given for unwanted changes, people can eventually learn to increase or decrease their heart rate at will. Neurofeedback uses this principle to try to give people some control over their brain waves by using the output from EEG to illustrate brain activity.

EEG

Our patterns of brain waves change all the time, depending on what we are doing. These patterns are measured by electroencephalography (almost always shortened to EEG). EEG records the electrical activity of the brain via electrodes that are glued to the scalp. Although it may look and sound alarming, an EEG is a short and painless procedure, with the only downside being the lumps of blue glue that you may find in your hair for a few days afterwards. Most people with epilepsy will be familiar with an EEG, as it is one of the very first diagnostic tests a doctor will order when they suspect someone may have had an epileptic seizure. Doctors have named some of the waves that an EEG detects after letters in the Greek alphabet. Alpha waves are oscillations in the frequency range of 8 to

12 cycles per second. These are normally associated with drowsiness and relaxation. They also happen automatically when you close your eyes. A beta wave or rhythm is used to describe activity in the next band of frequency, between 12 to 30 cycles per second. Beta waves can be associated with active concentration and also anxious ruminations. Delta waves are long and slow and are normally picked up by an EEG during deep sleep. Theta waves are also slower than alpha waves and are normally seen in children. Too much theta activity in adults can sometimes be a sign that something is wrong. However theta waves are also associated with some forms of meditation (see Chapter 10).

In addition to detecting normal changes in brain rhythms associated with everyday activities, an EEG can also detect abnormal patterns of brain waves. Some of the abnormal patterns that are most frequently associated with epilepsy are called epileptiform activity. Epileptiform activity looks like fast, synchronized wave patterns on the EEG. In some people with epilepsy, these abnormalities can be seen on an EEG even when someone is not having a seizure. In others, the brain waves look normal between seizures. In some cases, epileptiform abnormalities may only be picked up by a few electrodes that are all close to each other. If that is the case then it may be that just a small area of the brain is prone to seizures. If epileptiform abnormalities are seen synchronously throughout the entire brain, and this pattern is picked up by most of the electrodes on the EEG, then this suggests the individual may have a generalized epilepsy syndrome. People with focal epilepsy can have generalized seizures (where most of the brain is involved) but these are more likely to be secondary generalized seizures: seizures that begin in one small area of the brain and then spread to the rest of the brain causing a generalized convulsion.

It takes many years to learn to interpret an EEG and for most of us an EEG output just looks like rows of wiggly lines. However, in neurofeedback programmes the EEG lines are converted into a real-time display that everyone can understand. Sometimes this might be a video game similar to snakes and ladders where progression across the board is possible when the desired EEG patterns are present, but a snake may appear when the rhythms begin to deviate from this. Other feedback techniques may involve sounds or lights that turn on when particular patterns of brain activity are detected by the system.

What's the evidence?

Since 1970, there have been over 60 scientific studies published that have looked at whether neurofeedback can be helpful in controlling seizures for people with epilepsy. Many of these papers report encouraging findings, but the numbers of people in each of the individual studies have generally been too small for us to be really sure that neurofeedback is an effective treatment. One way around this problem is to use a meta-analysis. In a meta-analysis, researchers examine all the scientific reports on a given treatment and pool the data from as many people as they can, creating one giant study. This gives us information about how a treatment has worked for a much larger group of people than can ever be reported in any single study.

Texas research

In 2009, researchers from Texas published a meta-analysis of all the studies that have looked at neurofeedback in epilepsy. Although the researchers had to disregard the data from many of the studies, as not enough information was available on the people who took part, they found ten high quality studies which provided enough information for the participants to be included in a meta-analysis. All of the participants in these studies had seizures that were not fully controlled by medication. Three-quarters of the people who tried neurofeedback reported fewer weekly seizures following the sessions. The Texan researchers concluded that neurofeedback was an effective treatment for epilepsy. This finding from the meta-analysis is particularly impressive, given that all of the people who took part had seizures that were not fully controlled with anti-epileptic drugs.

Will it work for you?

Although the findings from studies of neurofeedback are encouraging there are still many gaps in our knowledge. For example, it is not known how long the effects last and there is an ongoing debate between scientists regarding the best EEG rhythm to train. A typical 'course' of neurofeedback training for epilepsy may involve two one-hour sessions every week, for three months or more. This will involve a considerable personal commitment of both time and money. It is very difficult to get neurofeedback on the NHS in the UK unless it is part of a research project at one of the university hospitals. There are numerous private providers of neurofeedback training, but packages of 20 sessions may cost upwards of £1000, placing this therapy out of reach for many people. It is also worth bearing in mind that many of the most prominent private providers of neurofeedback in the UK are not epilepsy specialists but provide the service for a variety of reasons, including personal and spiritual development. If you do wish to pursue neurofeedback as a complementary therapy for epilepsy it is important that you find a practitioner who is knowledgeable about epilepsy and aware of the latest clinical research in this area to ensure that you gain maximum benefit from the treatment.

17

Music therapy

Music affects the brain in many ways. Regardless of any talent or interest in music, our brains appear to be hardwired to tune into the underlying rhythms of music very quickly and we often react physically to this beat, moving in time to the music. Keen runners use this phenomenon to create 'running playlists' on their MP3 players to help them keep up their pace when they are running, but it also often happens unconsciously. In shopping centres or in the street, we may become aware that we are walking or moving in time to music that, moments before, we were not even aware was playing in the background. Retailers have reportedly used our unconscious tendencies to 'move to the beat' to speed up, or slow down, the movement of shoppers through supermarkets.

But music is more than just a beat. Musical melodies are processed in a different part of the brain, and the right temporal lobe in particular 'lights up' when people listen to music in an MRI scanner. The temporal lobes are also involved in the emotional reactions we have when we listen to music. The auditory nerve, the pathway that the brain uses to interpret external sounds, is linked in to a collection of closely connected parts of the brain called the limbic system. The structures that make up the limbic system are involved in memory and the processing of emotions. Even music without words can have a strong effect on our emotions. Uplifting tunes can make us feel euphoric, other stirring compositions can reduce people to tears. People who experience strong emotional reactions to music are often unable to say why the music has moved them; much of our emotional response appears to be unconscious, often labelled 'a gut response'. Adding meaningful lyrics to these tunes can make for a strong cathartic experience. Lovelorn teenagers (and some of us a good deal older) do not need a music therapist to introduce us to the powerful effects of 'sad songs' in helping us to process painful emotions.

Although music therapy only became formalized as a therapeutic approach in the twentieth century, the therapeutic effects of listening to music have been written about for millennia. Plato devoted much time to the role that music, rhythm and harmonies should play in his vision of 'The Republic', and wrote eloquently about the way in which music can be used to both rouse and soothe the masses.

Today, music therapists use music as part of a wider therapeutic relationship to help people with a wide variety of physical and psychological problems. Music can be used as an effective relaxation technique and can provide therapists with a way in, helping people express feelings and emotions that they find it difficult to articulate in other ways. Familiar tunes can often elicit a response even in people with severe dementia who do not respond to any other social approaches and, as a result, music therapy is now part of the therapeutic package in many care homes for the elderly. Those of you who love music will not be surprised to learn that numerous studies have suggested that several chemicals that play large a part in our experience of pleasure and reward with the brain, such as endorphins, endocannabinoids, dopamine and nitric oxide, also play an important role in the musical experience.

Music and epilepsy

Some types of epileptic seizure have strong associations with music. Parts of the limbic system become very epileptogenic (that is, prone to cause seizures) when they become damaged. For some people, music can either trigger a seizure or the experience of music can become part of the seizure. Musicogenic seizures are seizures that are triggered by hearing music. They are a kind of reflex epilepsy (see Chapter 4). Within this minority, people with pure musicogenic seizures, seizures that are only triggered by music, are even more unusual. Four out of five people with musicogenic epilepsy will experience at least some spontaneous seizures that are not triggered by music.

For some people with pure musicogenic epilepsy, their seizures may be triggered by a very specific piece of music.

French music lover

In 2003, French doctors reported the case of a 39-year-old woman who was a music lover and a singer. Her seizures were triggered whenever she heard Andrea Bocelli sing 'Con te partirò'. Unfortunately, it was a piece of music she really liked. Although she could avoid this particular tune relatively easily, at other times her seizures were triggered by supermarket music or mobile phone ringtones; sounds that surrounded her in every-day life and over which she had little control. Her EEG studies showed that the seizures were starting in the right temporal lobe. Interestingly, she did not have a seizure if she only heard the tune through her right ear.

Musical hallucinations can also form part of seizure and for some it may be the only clear manifestation that something is wrong. People may hear a particular tune very clearly and may have an impression that music is playing somewhere nearby, in a place that is difficult to pin down. We have all experienced the irritating phenomenon of songs that we cannot get out of our head, but for some people during a seizure, they really can 'hear' these songs in their head, sometimes playing very loudly, as the musical circuitry within the brain begins to fire up of its own accord. Interestingly, carbamazepine, one of the most commonly employed anti-epileptic medications, seems to have a particularly potent effect in preventing these kinds of seizures. There is also some evidence that taking carbamazepine may influence the perception of pitch in people with musical training.

Two young Japanese musicians

Doctors in Japan reported the cases of two young musicians aged 7 and 14 who noticed after they started to take carbamazepine that when they played the piano it sounded a half pitch lower than it should. When they stopped taking the drug, their perceptions of pitch returned to normal.

It seems probable that the changes in pitch perception associated with carbamazepine are more widespread than the occasional case studies in the medical literature suggest, but this goes unnoticed in the majority of people with epilepsy who are not musically trained. However, this peculiarly subtle effect of carbamazepine should be monitored in people who need perfect pitch perception for their work or musical pursuits.

The Mozart effect

Although music can trigger seizures in a minority of people with epilepsy, exposure to certain types of music may have a therapeutic effect in reducing seizure frequencies in many more. The 'Mozart effect' is a broad term that has come to encompass a wide range of purported beneficial effects of listening to some of Mozart's compositions. These range from apparent increases in childhood IQ to a speeding up of sewage processing in microbes subjected to arias from *The Magic Flute*. The Mozart effect originated from a paper published in 1993 in *Nature*, one of the most highly regarded scientific journals in the world. In the original study, 36 students completed abstract reasoning tasks, first after listening to Mozart, then again after listening to a relaxation tape and finally following a period of silence. The students obtained the highest scores on the tasks after they had listened to the Mozart piece. Although the improved cognitive processing only appears to last about ten minutes, simplistic press reporting and a number of commercially driven distortions of the original work over the subsequent years mean that the idea that listening to Mozart will somehow make you cleverer has permeated deep into the middle-class psyche. The original researchers have gone to great lengths to point out the limitations of their work, but nevertheless, the idea that listening to Mozart can somehow improve your IQ remains popular. However, while the jury may be out when it comes to the effects of listening to Mozart and an improvement in IQ, there is an increasing body of evidence to suggest that it may have a beneficial effect in epilepsy.

Certain Mozart pieces appear to influence the brain activity as measured by an EEG. In 1998, researchers in the USA played Mozart's sonata for two pianos in D major (K.448) to 29 people with epilepsy, who were being monitored via EEG. Significant decreases in epileptiform abnormalities (abnormal brain waves) were seen on the EEG in an impressive 23 out of the 29 cases. Some of the people in this study were in a coma or in status epilepticus and had no overt signs of awareness that the music was even playing. In one person who was in a coma, the amount of epileptic activity on their EEG decreased from 62 to 21 per cent when the music was played. In a further study the researchers found that the same piece of music led to a reduction in both EEG abnormalities and clinical seizures over a 24-hour period when people with epilepsy listened to Mozart for ten minutes every hour when they were awake.

Three studies

On the other side of the world, researchers in Taiwan also found that four out of five children who listened to the same Mozart piece had a reduction in abnormal EEG activity. In that study, it was the children who had generalized epilepsy who showed the most improvements. In another case, a man with gelastic seizures (seizures that manifest themselves as spontaneous bouts of giggling or laughing, without any external trigger for the mirth or subjective feelings of happiness) listened to Mozart on a daily basis and experienced a significant reduction in his seizures as a result. In 2011, Taiwanese researchers looked at the effects of listening to Mozart once a day before bedtime for six months in a group of 11 children whose epilepsy was not well controlled, despite the fact that they had taken at least two anti-epileptic drugs for at least a year. The results were remarkable. Two of the children were seizure-free and a further six had a very good response to the treatment, with a greater than 50 per cent reduction in the number of seizures they experienced after six months of listening to Mozart K.448.

Researchers have tried to analyze the ways in which this particular Mozart sonata is distinct from other pieces of music that do not produce this effect. In music theory, periodicity is a term given to the predictability that gives rise to expectations about what is coming next. The epilepsy researchers concluded that the complex repetitions and predictable patterns of scales within the Mozart piece gave it a long-term periodicity. This engages many areas of the brain in encoding the patterns and recognizing and predicting what will come next. Somehow, this complex activity seems to resonate within the brain and change the EEG rhythms as a result. Although many other composers, particularly classical composers, use periodicity in their work, it appears to be long-term periodicity associated with this particular Mozart piece that has the most impact on EEG measures.

Will it work for you?

Music therapy should probably be avoided by anyone with musicogenic seizures, i.e. seizures triggered by music. Although some have used gradual and controlled exposure to these very specific triggers to try to build up a kind of resistance, the few attempts that have been reported in the medical literature have not given much ground for optimism in pursuing such an approach.

Music therapy, in its widest sense, may be effective in helping people with epilepsy confront some of the difficult social and stigmatizing aspects of the condition that they may find it difficult to express in more conventional forums. It may be particularly useful for children or adults with learning disabilities or other difficulties in communication. However, there remains a dearth of rigorous scientific studies evaluating the effectiveness of music therapy in epilepsy as a whole.

In terms of seizure control there is a converging body of evidence to suggest that the 'Mozart effect' may be effective in reducing EEG abnormalities, particularly widespread generalized discharges. Recent work has also suggested that listening to Mozart K.448, once a day before bedtime, may result in a reduction in seizures. Although this has yet to be proven helpful in a controlled trial of adults with epilepsy, the results from the small study of children are very encouraging. In terms of trying this as an add-on therapy, it seems as if there is very little to lose (except perhaps a few pounds for the CD if you do not already own it), and it does have the potential for quite significant gains, particularly for controlling generalized seizures.

18

Pet therapy

Pet therapy is not a treatment in the way that many of the therapies discussed so far have been. Many people, particularly those who are already pet owners, believe that their pets enhance their lives immeasurably and would not be without them. Scientists have started to look to see whether owning a pet actually has a measurable impact on well-being and health. Almost all of the work that has been completed to date has looked at the effects on health of owning dogs and cats, since these are the most popular domestic pets in Western societies.

One of the biggest problems with this approach is that the people who take part in these studies inevitably already own a pet. Since 'A dog is for life and not just for Christmas', it is not possible to randomly allocate pets to people and take them away from others. Looking after a dog or cat will probably involve more than a decade of care and financial commitment. It stands to reason that people who have already made the decision to own a pet may already be different in important respects from those who have not chosen to share their home with an animal. These pre-existing differences may account for some of the findings attributed to the beneficial effects of pet ownership in the scientific literature.

What's the evidence?

Since, in the real world, it is not practical to randomly allocate pets to people, there are no randomized controlled trials of pet therapy for people with epilepsy. But the results from the studies that have been done with other illnesses may surprise you. In 2010, an American study of over 11,000 people found that dog owners did more exercise than people who did not own a dog and that, as a result, they tended to live longer. When they compared the beneficial effects of owning a cat compared to a dog, they concluded that it was the increased level of exercise, rather than the companionship of an animal, that was associated with the increase in life expectancy.

Canadian scientists found that owning a pet also tended to keep older people living independently for longer and that the pets helped them to maintain their social life. But when they too came to look at whether pet owners were generally healthier or happier they could not find any differences between people who had pets and those that did not.

In 2005, doctors in Australia looked at how often two groups of older people, with and without pets, visited their GPs over the course of a year. In this study, people who owned pets were more depressed than those who didn't and also had poorer physical health. The doctors concluded that pet ownership conferred no clear health benefits for older people.

Likewise in Scandinavia, pet ownership has not been universally associated with positive health benefits. In Finland, a study of over 21,000 people found that pet ownership was associated with poor, rather than good, perceived health. Over the border in Sweden, researchers looked at the effects of owning a pet in over 43,000 people. They found that although pet owners were more likely to be more physically active than people without pets, they were also more likely to complain about general aches and pains, including headaches.

In Belfast, a survey study of 193 people with chronic fatigue syndrome found that pet owners believed that their pets had the potential to enhance their quality of life. However, they did not differ from their fellow sufferers who did not own pets on any of the measures of general health that the researchers used, and the complaints of fatigue were the same in both groups.

The upshot of all these studies seems to suggest that people who own pets certainly feel that they enrich their lives. People who own dogs generally get more beneficial exercise, to the point that it may even increase their life expectancy, than those who do not. In this respect a dog is rather like a personal trainer. Instead of barking motivational instructions at you, dogs that are under-exercised get bored and frustrated and tend to become a nuisance around the house, chewing toys, shoes and furniture. Thus, they make it more likely that you will go out every day and at least get some fresh air, if not moderate exercise. Living with a dog also helps some people to regulate their own sleep–wake cycle, as dogs tend to get up regularly in the mornings and need to be let out to relieve themselves, preventing long lie-ins and gradual shifts in the day–night pattern in their owners, shifts that can be detrimental for seizure control for some people with epilepsy.

However, beyond these benefits and those of exercise, there has been a distinct lack of measurable health benefits from the companionship of an animal. It is striking that these findings are fairly consistent across the developed world, from Scandinavia to Australia, particularly given the cultural differences in attitudes toward pets in each country. It is impossible to tease apart cause from effect in these studies, but the results do suggest that the companionship of an animal, by itself, has little impact on health.

Pets and stress reduction

Although owning a pet does not appear to have any specific health benefits, there is a small body of evidence to suggest that it may be helpful in reducing stress. Stroking a pet releases oxytocin, in both the person stroking and the animal. Oxytocin is a hormone that promotes bonding and is associated with feelings of well-being and tranquillity. Much of this work has been completed with people who suffer from high blood pressure and cardiovascular problems. People who own pets tend to have lower blood pressure than those who do not and they are also more likely to survive a heart attack. In one experiment, researchers put people in a stressful situation by placing their hand in cold water while making them solve difficult mental arithmetic problems. Interestingly, people showed much less stress on physiological measures if their pet was in the room with them when this happened. Having a spouse in the room actually increased the levels of stress, probably because the person did not want to look foolish struggling with the maths test in front of their partner. This study neatly illustrates the advantages of social support from a pet; it is not judgmental.

Dogs and epilepsy

The evidence suggests that pet ownership, in and of itself, will probably not have an appreciable effect on the frequency of seizures in people who have epilepsy, although possible spin-offs, including increased exercise and reduced levels of stress, may be beneficial for some. However, dogs may be able to play other helpful roles for people with epilepsy.

Interest in 'seizure alert dogs' began in the 1990s. Seizure alert dogs are animals that appear to sense that their owner is going to have a seizure, well before the person themselves is aware of any changes. These dogs exhibit a change in their own behaviour, in response to the changes they detect in their owner. If the owner can recognize these changes, the dog can be used as a 'warning system', letting the person know that a seizure is coming, and giving them time to make themselves safe. Once a dog has shown some sensitivity to pre-seizure changes they perceive in their owner, they can be trained to carry out very explicit actions to alert their owner of the impending seizure.

This kind of training is very intensive and necessitates a very close relationship between the dog and its owner, similar to that required by guide dogs for the blind. The dog must be focused on the needs of its owner at all times to the exclusion of other distractions. This is often not possible in a domestic situation with a family pet. In addition, it takes a long time to build up this kind of relationship, and at the end there is no guarantee that the dog will be able to sense any changes in its owner prior to the seizure. In reality, it seems that a seizure alert dog may represent a rare, serendipitous relationship, rather than one that can be created at will, no matter how rigorous the training.

The mechanisms by which a dog may be able to sense a seizure before it happens are unknown. Some have suggested that these dogs actually sense increasing levels of emotional distress in their owners and that the subsequent 'seizure' isn't an epileptic seizure but a non-epileptic attack (something that looks like an epileptic seizure, but has a psychological basis).

While one cannot reliably train a dog to predict when a seizure is about to happen, it is far easier to teach a dog to recognize a seizure in their owner when it does occur. Some dogs can, therefore, be trained to be of practical help for some people with epilepsy.

Heidi

One example of this is Heidi, who developed epilepsy in her late teens. She keeps a laminated card in her pocket when she goes shopping. If she has a seizure, her dog, Charley, recognizes the abnormal behaviour, removes the card from her pocket and takes it to the nearest person. The card gives details of Heidi's typical seizures, including how long they usually last, and has a phone number to call to alert her parents as to what has happened. Although she cheerfully admits it can go wrong, Heidi knows that Charley's actions have prevented unnecessary 999 calls and time-consuming trips to the A&E department when concerned members of the public have panicked at the sight of a young woman convulsing. Charley wears a high visibility 'assistant dog' jacket when she accompanies Heidi shopping.

Generally, the larger retail outlets are becoming more aware of the variety of the 'assistant' roles dogs can play for people with a wide range of needs and, increasingly, few restrict entrance to just guide dogs for the blind.

Will it work for you?

Pet therapies are not designed for specific seizure types. There is no evidence that owning a pet will decrease the number of seizures you experience. Having a dog may provide you with the motivation to exercise, and stroking and interacting with pets may reduce your stress levels. Both exercise and stress reduction may make it less likely that you have a seizure. However, owning a pet is a big personal commitment, in time, money and emotion. The decision to get a pet should be based on a careful consideration of how it will fit into your current lifestyle. Any anticipated effects on health should be viewed as a bonus rather than the *raison d'être* of the pet.

19

Conclusions

The preceding chapters have reviewed both the scientific under-pinnings and the clinical evidence for numerous alternative and complementary treatments that are offered for epilepsy today. As a whole, the therapies can be divided into three broad groups:

- therapies that have been specifically designed to treat epilepsy;
- therapies based on unproven ideas;
- therapies that may have an indirect benefit on seizures.

Therapies that have been specifically designed to treat epilepsy

The scientific rationale behind these treatments is usually based on an understanding of how and why seizures happen, and scientists have used this knowledge to try and modify a pattern to make a seizure less likely to occur. The development of light therapy for epilepsy is a good example of such an approach. It comes from our current understanding of the way in which brain chemistry responds to light and how it influences seizure thresholds, particularly in people with temporal lobe epilepsy. Neurofeedback is another good example of such an approach and has its foundations firmly set in observable abnormal brain waves that can be modified and trained.

Therapies based on unproven ideas

It is unsurprising that the treatment approaches that have sound theoretical underpinnings, consistent with what we know about epilepsy and the natural laws of science, tend to show better results in clinical trials of their effectiveness in reducing seizures than the second group of treatment approaches based on hypothetical, unproven scientific foundations. In the case of some, such as homoeopathy, the scientific foundation of the approach (infinite dilution) has been disproved by subsequent discoveries in science (the existence of molecules). Likewise, scientific advances in physiology and biology have made a nonsense of the late eighteenth century fad to attribute all illnesses to a single physical cause, such as a misaligned spine.

Treatment approaches based on at best hypothetical, and at worst scientifically antithetical, foundations are often grounded in a holistic view of disease, where epilepsy is just one manifestation of an imbalance within the human system. Rebalancing this system may be attempted by physical means, for example in chiropractic care, or chemically, for example homoeopathy. Many of these approaches were developed in the late nineteenth and early twentieth century and the originators often incorporated an additional spiritual or supernatural element to the healing, invoking the concept of a life force beyond the physical body. These ideas are similar to the ancient philosophical bases of Ayurveda and TCM. In many ways, this philosophical approach resulted in the development of generic treatments in search of diseases rather than vice versa. As such, these approaches continue to be used for a wide variety of conditions, not just epilepsy.

In some of the therapies available today, the rationale behind the healing borders on the magical. In craniosacral therapy, for example, some practitioners claim not only to be able to sense abnormal brain rhythms and pathology, but also the capacity to manipulate them through the skull. If this were possible, the human fingertips would have the combined power of both an MRI scan and the best EEG technology. Unfortunately, but perhaps unsurprisingly, such feats have not been proven. On the whole, there is little or no reliable clinical evidence to suggest that these approaches are successful in reducing seizures. An absence of evidence that something works is not, in itself, evidence that it does not work., However, if something does work, it is relatively easy to prove. Many of the practitioners of these therapies argue that the primary reason for the lack of scientific evidence is that they have no funds to conduct rigorous clinical trials. It becomes a circular argument. The reason they find it hard to find funding for a trial is that organisations that allocate research grants usually base their decisions on a detailed scrutiny of the scientific underpinnings of new treatments. If it does not look like it might work on paper, funding organizations are unlikely to devote their precious, scarce funds to proving it. And so these therapies continue to be offered in the absence of any real evidence that they work, save for the occasional anecdotal report of improvement in someone. In the age of the internet, these highly personal tales of a miracle response spread fast and wide and can offer false hope to many who have reached the end of the road in conventional treatments.

Every new generation thinks that now we finally know the truth, dismissing old archaic ideas and embracing the new. However, any student of scientific history will tell you that what we actually 'know' at any one time is just a working model of the way we think the world works. This model may, at any time, be surpassed by an entirely different 'knowledge'. While we know much about how the body works, there is much more that we do not know. Genetic studies are beginning to reveal that single deletions in the genetic code may be associated with a variety of apparently disparate symptoms. Recent work has linked one small kink in the genetic code to very mild, but nevertheless consistent, anomalies in the shape of someone's face and the propensity to have seizures. Biological systems that we have until very recently thought of as separate, may be governed by the same parts of our genetic code.

We are only just beginning to scratch the surface of the complex way that the mind interacts with the body. Time and time again, studies show that psychological factors are important in a large number of apparently physical conditions ranging from heart disease to cancer. The placebo effect (discussed in Chapter 2) is a fascinating example of this. We really do not know how it works and some doctors are keen to dismiss it. But they are missing a trick. The placebo is something that works. It works for epilepsy. It should not work, we cannot explain it and it does not work for everyone. But for some, it does. It seems probable that at least some of the holistic therapies are also tapping into this process. So, while it is highly unlikely that they will be effective in controlling seizures for the reasons they give, some of these therapies may still have a beneficial effect for some people. Conventional doctors dismiss this important extra dimension of psychological factors in healing, to the detriment of their patients.

Therapies that may have an indirect benefit on seizures

The third group of treatments discussed in this book are therapies that may have an indirect benefit for people with epilepsy. Anything that reduces stress may make a seizure less likely. This is likely to be highly individual. Some may find a massage with essential oils very effective, while others may feel embarrassed and tense during the procedure. Similarly, a pet can be a great source of relaxation or of stress, depending on your relationship with the animal. The comprehensive neurobehavioural approach capitalizes on the relationship between stress and seizures, and if followed closely may help an individual gain a greater understanding and possibly even control over the relationship between stress and their seizures.

If you do not try, you will never know

While there is often little or no evidence to support many of the complementary and alternative therapies for epilepsy reviewed in this book, there remains much you can try. A healthy diet, regular exercise, aromatherapy, neurofeedback, light therapy, the Mozart effect and the comprehensive neurobehavioural approach all have something to commend them in epilepsy, as does anything that may reduce the stress in your life. Some have argued that there is no such thing as alternative medicine, only medicine that works and medicine that does not. If you do not try, you will never know whether a new approach will work for you.

Useful addresses

The resources listed here give more detailed information on many of the issues and studies described in this book.

General information

Epilepsy Action (previously **British Epilepsy Association**)
New Anstey House
Gate Way Drive
Yeadon, Leeds LS19 7XY
Tel.: 0113 210 8800
Freephone helpline: 0808 800 5050
Text helpline: 07797 805 390
Website: www.epilepsy.org.uk

Epilepsy Society (previously **National Society for Epilepsy**)
Chesham Lane
Chalfont St Peter
Gerrards Cross
Bucks SL9 0RJ
Tel.: 01494 601 300
Helpline: 01494 601 400 (10 a.m. to 4 p.m., Monday to Friday)
Website: www.epilepsysociety.org.uk

The International League against Epilepsy (ILAE)
342 North Main Street
West Hartford
CT 06117-2507, USA
Tel.: 860.586.7547
Website: www.ilae-epilepsy.org
Provides up-to-date information about the current terminology and concepts used to classify epilepsy syndromes and seizures.

Medicines and Healthcare products Regulatory Agency (MHRA)
151 Buckingham Palace Road
London SW1W 9SZ
Tel.: 020 3080 6000 (Central Enquiry Point: 9 a.m. to 5 p.m., Monday to Friday)
Website: www.mhra.gov.uk
Regulates licensed herbal medicines.

Useful websites

On diet

General information about health and diet can be found on the UK's **National Health Service** website: www.nhs.uk/LiveWell/Healthyeating. In the United States the **Office of Dietary Supplements**, part of the US National Institutes of Health organization, also provides reliable, science-based facts on dietary supplements. See www.ods.od.nih.gov.

On evidence-based medicine

Information on this and the Cochrane Collaboration can be accessed from the **Cochrane Library** (www.thecochranelibrary.com). The library holds more than 80 reviews of epilepsy treatments, all of which are available to download and read, free of charge. Each report also has a plain-language summary, written for people without any specialist scientific or medical background. In addition, **Sense about Science** is a British charity that promotes the public understanding of science, and also respect for scientific evidence and good science: www.senseaboutscience.org.

Seizure diaries

You can download blank seizure diary templates from the internet (e.g. www.epilepsy.org.uk). The site <www.epilepsy.com> also provides an online diary application called 'My Epilepsy Diary' which has space for all kinds of information, and you can even print out useful summaries to take to your doctor for each appointment. There is now a version of 'My Epilepsy Diary' for the MP3 player, smartphone and tablet PC.

Other useful websites

The Andrews/Reiter Epilepsy Research Program Inc. in California provides information on the comprehensive neurobehavioural approach to epilepsy: www.andrewsreiter.com

Epilepsy.com is a comprehensive, interactive information site based in the USA: www.epilepsy.com

The Science and Technology Parliamentary Select Committee Sixth Report on complementary and alternative medicine, published in November 2000, may be accessed from: www.publications.parliament.uk/pa/ld199900/ldselect/ldsctech/123/12301.htm

The United States section of the **World Wildlife Fund** is organizing an awareness campaign on traditional Chinese medicine: www.worldwildlife.org/what/globalmarkets/wildlifetrade/traditional chinesemedicine.html

Further reading

On evidence-based medicine

The following books offer a broad and accessible overview of the importance of fair tests when it comes to looking at whether medicines work or not:

Goldacre, Dr Ben, *Bad Science*, Fourth Estate, London, 2008.
Singh, Simon, and Ernst, Edzard, *Trick or Treatment? Alternative medicine on trial.* Corgi, London, 2009.

Other useful resources

Details of how to obtain the following book can be found at www.andrews reiter.com:

Reiter, J. M., Andrews, D., and Janis, C., *Taking Control of Your Epilepsy: A workbook for patients and professionals.* Basics, Santa Rosa, CA, 1987.

You can read more about aromatherapy and epilepsy and many other alternative and complementary treatments for epilepsy in the following book, edited by three professors who are among the most eminent epileptologists in the world:

Devinsky, Orrin, Schachter, Steven, and Pacia, Steven, *Complementary and Alternative Therapies for Epilepsy.* Demos Medical Publishing, New York, 2005.

In this textbook, over twenty complementary practitioners describe their experiences with alternative treatments, and the editors provide a balanced commentary on the evidence base for each approach.

Index